CHLORELLA

-Functional Food-

BY

STIG ARNE LEVIN

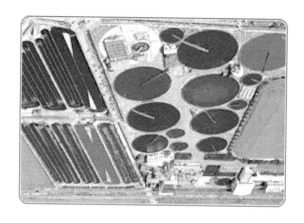

I sincerely thank my wife Birgitta, who has assisted me during my past 27 years of research with chlorella and how she has stimulated me in my work with this book about chlorella pyrenoidosa.

I am also inspired by Dr. Bernard Jensen, Dr. David Steenblock and Professor Randall Merchant from USA as well as having had possibilities to read their books about Chlorella. I also wish to thank Mr. Pascal Caussimon in France for his assistance making this book real. Also, I have made my research on chlorella during 27 years and learned a lot from people with different health problems having been taken care of and treated by physicians when eating chlorella pyrenoidosa.

Finally, I honor all people who lived in Nagasaki and Hiroshima, Japan, when the atom bomb was thrown at them and killed innocent people. May ICAN be able to help saving the world from nuclear weapon.

Warning: All material presented herein, is for information only and should not be interpreted as indication that Chlorella can or should be used to treat any disease or condition. This information is not intended to be as a prescription or as a replacement of medications prescribed by your physician in the treatment of any specific illness. The author assumes no responsibility for any adverse outcome or problem that occur if a person elects to use any of the information contained within this book.

Cover design: Caussimon Pascal, France

Contents

Preface

I'm sure we all want to feel physically and mentally fit as long as we live. Unfortunately, as a child, we did not learn how to prepare ourselves for the future in terms of nutrition, nor the knowledge of an appropriate lifestyle which could lead to a long life with good health.

With good health, I mean not only regular heart-beats and good bowel movements.

Good health also includes a positive attitude, hope, self-acceptance, creativity, job satisfaction, gratitude and ability to accept and to appreciate your fellow human beings. All this and more needed to make us feel real good. However, without the proper food and a proper lifestyle, nothing can work out of the above.

If you do not eat a proper, nutritious and balanced food, you cannot get mental and bodily balance. Our parents simply did not have the correct knowledge of nutrition and perhaps it was because, about 50 years ago, they thought the basic food was sufficient and could not be affected to such an extent by the development of the industrial society.

Since then, however, the diet has been depleted and the animals have been treated with hormones and antibiotics and otherwise contaminated. It has, in turn, contributed to the development of various cancerous diseases and other genetic influenced diseases such as allergy, depression, overweight and diabetes which have increasingly affected us. Not least there is an increased development of cardiovascular diseases.

At about 20 years of age, our body begins to age.

We produce less of the essential substances needed to keep the body as healthy and resilient as in the teenage years.

During our life, we often struggle to get along at work and to get better economy and higher status in society, while eating wrong and unhealthy food, exercising too rarely, smoking, consuming too much alcohol and drinking too little of clean water.
Many of us have severe sleep problems, not least women, which can cause a decaying effect on the body, both physically and mentally.

We put ourselves in imbalance!

The body has an innate intelligence. Your own body is the best doctor. It is daily exposed to a variety of harmful environmental hazards and improper lifestyle, but has the ability to cure itself. No person can artificially do what the body itself accomplishes all the time. **This is called natural healing.**

We contribute to impaired health by weakening our own immune system, which will provide a good protection against attacks of foreign bacteria and damage through existing heavy metals and bacteria in our environment.
Sometimes you can eat a salad occasionally, sweat at a gym more or less regularly, play golf and maybe jog during hot seasons and take a cure with some multivitamin.
But, that's not easy now.
Because body and soul work together, it may be primarily to think and act healthy in order to help your body work better.
A well balanced psyche can be easily achieved by means of a good physical health. One can say that the body is the shadow of the mind.

But we need beneficial stimulus for the body to balance and thereby work better.

OUR DAILY FOOD AND OUR FOOD PRODUCTION

Many people suffer from fatigue, depression, stress, allergies, stomach upset, pain, unbalanced metabolism and reduced body functions. In the daily diet is often lacking some important nutrients while constantly exposing us to air pollution, pesticides, dyestuff and other chemical additives in food and water.

These harmful and for our body, completely foreign chemicals and heavy metals, propagate in our organism and cause devastating health problems when they exceed the body's tolerance level.

This, in turn, leads to a weakened immune system, which means that the body is not able to defend itself against causes ranging from mild to severe allergies, genetic, physical and mental illnesses and cancer.

We can change by giving our body additional nutrients by ingesting such as Chlorella pyrenoidosa, that our body genetically recognizes and thus can be effectively addressed.

Not least important is that chlorella pyrenoidosa also helps cleanse the body from foreign, harmful sub-stances, heavy metals and foreign bacteria. Important is of course also to do daily exercise and eating a balanced, nutritious and healthy diet.

Fluid intake of at least 2 liters of clean water and good sleep are also important factors that contribute to a better physical balance.

All humans have a need of a strong immune system in the fight against cancer, viruses, allergies, and other physical and mental illnesses.

100 years ago, our food that we consumed and produced was of other quality than what we can eat and what we are consuming today.

I remember myself of the real and naturally produced milk, butter, cream and cheese as well as the much better nutritious value of vegetables in those days.

Today and since at least 50 years, our food is changed and have become less nutritious because of the way it is produced in order to keep it better conserved and to make more money of it.

That is why we are more vulnerable, experiencing more of various diseases, symptoms, fatigues, depressions, and other problems.

Cancer is increasing as well as diabetes 2, birth of children having a lot of genetic problems like brain cancer, diabetes 1 and many other problems.

The question is who is going to take care of these problems and the developments for us humans. The answer to this should be: **ourselves**.

A great thing is to study how the Aztecs and the Hunza People lived in past time. Their daily life style and what they ate.

This way, we would learn how to and what to eat to stay healthy and live happily longer.

It is important to be able to see the need for a healthy lifestyle and for balanced food regimen in our lives.

I think it is very important to listen to your own body and what it has to say. When you know what your body needs, you can easier take care of it and make what it needs to get better.

Fortunately, it's never too late to do something about it.

First, try to listen to your own body and think logically.

Our body does not just tell us when it is in good condition, but it is immediately reminded of the opposite when it is bad. You may experience aches and discomfort which is the cause of imbalance as it is important to pay attention to and learn the reason for the more effective treatment of the problems.

You can help your body to get better balance by changing lifestyle, eat more nutritious "live foods," avoiding junk food, planning your "everyday" life, and work better, exercising regularly and trying to avoid too much of stress.

To allow your body to daily get rid of toxic material, while providing it a balanced nutritional and complete feed, is a crucial step towards better health.

One of the many tools and stimulus for better health balance that has existed since the end of World War II, is Chlorella pyrenoidosa, which today is the most studied and best-selling functional food in Japan, where it has already since long, been appointed functional food Nr. 1.

Today, other parts of the world have learned about Chlorella and it is used as food in many other countries, medically and as healthy food for every day use to many health loving people.

This little green micro alga is over 3,5 billions years old (pre-Cambrian) and became the first time known for humanity in 1890 when chlorella was found outside the Dutch coast by a micro-biologist named M.W. Beijerinck who began research.

I have tried to gather information about chlorella from 128 years of research.

By this book, I want to explain why chlorella is eaten daily by more than 20-25 million people around the world as a supplement to the daily diet and also as an ingredient in many food dishes.

Chlorella is no drug but a natural and nutritionally complete food such as "functional" food that can be eaten every day by everyone, old and young and not to forget how useful it is for pregnant women. Chlorella also provides nutrition to healthcare professionals in many countries.

Basic information in this book about chlorella is derived from a variety of clinical trials and treatment methods that have been done for more than a hundred years, and are yet used by doctors, researchers and therapists in general and alternative careers.

We need to improve our physical and mental balance!

Nevertheless, it is never too late to start caring for the body, our most important capital, if the goal is to acquire physical and mental balance, better health and thus better quality of life.

This means that you primarily seek to detoxify the body from toxic substances and prevent malnutrition by eating proper and healthy foods.

Twenty-seven years ago, I was given the tip of a French doctor to regularly eat chlorella pyrenoidosa in order to detoxify my body while giving myself a well balanced, complete nutrition in 100% natural form from nature.

The reason for my visit to a doctor, was to seek help for various problems that I acquired due to improper lifestyles over the years, as well as for my enlarged prostate organ that had given me a lot of problems.

Today, we call this condition "burned-out". Chlorella, with its nutrient richness and ability to detoxify my body, would give my body better physical and mental balance.

During the first three weeks of 3-5 grams chlorella pyrenoidosa per day, I gradually began to feel changes in my body. I was having my old energy and normal vitality back again.

My prostate problem disappeared completely when eating chlorella, as this organ is in need of the mineral zinc in order to function well.
My bowel system should work better than before, which I understood was assisting my body to both feel and become much healthier.
After three months intake of 3 grams per day of chlorella pyrenoidosa, I felt in a much better shape both body and soul. Previous symptoms had disappeared altogether.
I have been able to maintain my improved body balance and harmonious feeling, not least because I gradually changed my lifestyle and continued my daily intake of chlorella pyrenoidosa.

How to explain this positive reaction?
The body recognizes and quickly and effectively absorbs chlorella's natural nutritions that include vitamins, minerals, amino acids, fatty acids, RNA DNA, chlorophyll, xanthophyll and chlorella growth factor (CGF).
The detoxification process begins immediately with the assistance of chlorophyll and another active substance in chlorella's cell wall, *Sporopollenin*.
Sporopollenin contained in the middle layer of Chlorella's cell wall, causes heavy metals and foreign body bacteria to pass through the intestinal tract and

other excretory agents and finally is emptied from the body by bowel movements.
The immune system is gaining stimulus and the body begins to feel better and get more balance.

Algae

Nature has a huge selection of plants that can provide us with valuable raw materials for the manufacture of nutrients and medicines. For a long time, scientific research has been going on to investigated what the plant kingdom and the fauna have to offer of healing substances and important nutrients.
But it is still insufficient. More studies and research would be needed to solve more issues regarding nature's assets.
Since the 1920s, the pharmaceutical industry has put much efforts to isolate vitamins and other substances for synthetic production.
Synthetic substances can be patented and thus earn a lot of money for the producers.
However, it Is very important to understand that it is healthier and more useful to eat a nutrition, that comes 100% pure from nature, than to eat laboratory-based dietary supplements.
Chlorella pyrenoidosa is the plant that has showed the greatest interest in science due to its potential health promoting properties. Research with chlorella has been going on since 128 years, beginning in 1890. Chlorella, other green and blue/green algae, have had a significant role in the process of photosynthesis which is a prerequisite for all life.

Oxygen is namely being produced by photo-synthesis. This is a process involving plants like chlorella and other algae using their chloroplasts to capture energy from the sun. This is used to convert water and carbon dioxide to oxygen and sugar.

Some of this sugar is turned down to energy, while the rest is used for continuous growth.
The process means that carbon dioxide is taken from the atmosphere and a huge quantity of oxygen is released which in turn is needed for humans, animals and plants to live on our soil. Four-fifths of the earth's surface is covered with water and a substantial part of the world's resources are harvested from our oceans, lakes and rivers.

Perhaps it was due to high cultural values that we previously considered fish and shellfish as the most important feed in our streams and not to a greater extent had studied the value of plants as edible algae more closely.
In recent times, many new and remarkable foods have become available to many health conscious consumers worldwide.
Soy products such as tofu and tempeh, nutritional yeast and many traditional medicinal herbs are used today by those seeking a more natural and healthy living.

The most remarkable "new times" food that contain the highest concentration of holistic nutrition that exists in our world, are algae like chlorella, spirulina, dunaniella salina and scenedesmus.
In or near the Earth's watercourses there are more than 70,000 different species of algae mainly without roots, tribes, branches and leaves. Algae performs their own life functions such as reproduction.

They contain a variety of nutrients, vitamins, minerals, fatty acids, chlorophyll and xanthophyll and belong to the simplest living organisms.

Like other plants containing chlorophyll, the algae transform inorganic, chemical elements into organic substances using light energy and photosynthesis.

During the first billion years of existence, the atmosphere consisted of lethal gases such as ammonia and methane. It became the role of the green plants,(such as chlorella) to filter these deadly elements and make the environment adapt to flora and fauna.

Scientists estimate that algae are responsible for 90% of all photosynthesis that occur in the world. They form the first link in a series of organisms that make up our foodstuffs and grow everywhere, from the tropics to the polar regions.

Algae are elementary organisms that use sunlight to transform lifeless and non organic chemicals into living bio-organic tissues, which represents a higher form of existence.

Algae provide oxygen with water, which allows fish and other species to live in the world's oceans, rivers and lakes. They collect energy from the sun and store it in the form of food. Algae grow in an environment where there is enough water and you often see them on rocks, trees and even on the ground.

Water depth and temperature do not play a decisive role in the well-being of the algae. They can be found at a depth of 600 feet, some grow in snow and ice, others have been identified in hot springs with temperatures of 180 degrees or more.

For more than 100 years, researchers have studied algae and their organic functions and roles in our food chain.

Perhaps more than we know today, people and animals have used edible algae as food. Today, for example, is used a substance from an alga called Irish moss for chocolate milk, sauces and jams but also for tooth-paste and shampoo.
Another species, agar, is used in bakery products, sorbet, cheese, sweets and laxatives. Other species are used as dietary supplements in tablet or powder form.
   Some algae are more famous than others as being sources of vitamins, minerals, carbohydrates and pro-tein.

For a long time, algae have been eaten daily by millions of people in the Orient, partly as a dietary supplement in tablet or powder form, and partly as an ingredient in the daily diet.
   Today, more and more people, also in other parts of the world, have taken an interest in algae as an important element in daily food or as a healthy nu-tritional supplement and stimulus for the immune system. Green algae belongs to the most diverse group of algae with more than 7000 species growing in a variety of environments.
Like other plants, green algae contain chlorophyll, which they use to capture light energy as fuel for the production of sugar but different from other plants, they are primarily aquatic plants that produce their own nutrition.

Sea-algae

Under the concept of "sea-algae", there are a lot used in the manufacture of pharmaceuticals and cosmetics. The salt content of the sea has a certain influence on the nutritional content of the sea algae.

However, all sea algae contain a variety of egg-white as well as varying levels of iodine.

The high concentration of iodine is the one that most separates the sea algae from the freshwater algae, since the latter mentioned contain less of this mineral.

An excessive amount of iodine may adversely affect many people with overproducing thyroid problems and should therefore refrain from consuming sea algae.

Freshwater algae

Apart from containing a waste amount of iodine, freshwater algae as chlorella pyrenoidosa, contain important nutrients in extremely concentrated form for the body

In particular Chlorella is invaluable to the body as an important protein supplier, because we constantly need proteins as nutrition.

Remarkably and important to mention is Chlorella's growth. Under controlled growing conditions, it propagates 4 times in 16 to 20 hours and could thus be used as a good source of protein in the battle against world hunger, which is a catastrophic problem for millions of people. Chlorella's growth capacity is unique in its kind.

Eucaryotes

Eu comes from the Greek word for "real" and from the Greek karyon, which means core or cell. The cells of eukaryotes are the common genetic material of a cell nucleus enclosed by a cell membrane.

To eukaryotic organisms counts, people, animals, plants and some species of alga, such as Chlorella.

Eukaryotic algae also have "organs" for photosynthesis called chloroplasts whose chlorophyll content is concentrated and "stapled" to be able to utilize sunlight in the best and most efficient way.

Procaryotes
Contrary to eukaryotes, prokaryotes are more primitive organisms, whose cells contain neither a "real" nucleus or a cellular organ. Its genetic material in cytoplasm lies freely in the cell.
Cyanobacteria Spirulina and AFA, as other similar bacteria, count into prokaryotes and are often mistakenly referred to as blue algae or blue-green algae. Cyanobacteria are special bacteria that, like the plants, can perform photosynthesis.

Some spirulina bacteria are almost half a millimeter long, multicellular and spiral formed and grow in salty, hot water in subtropical areas such as Asia and Central Africa.

The most famous species is spirulina *platensis*, which is now also grown in large pools in Taiwan among some other countries under controlled conditions, where good quality is of utmost importance. This algae contain a lot of different active substances, of which 70% are egg-white substances as well as vitamins, minerals and traces substances.
The blue-green AFA bacteria grows close to wildly in Klamath Lake, Oregon, USA. It contains a significant amount of vitamin B12 (not being assimilated by human), chlorophyll and the protective pigment phycozyanin that claims to be able to protect against cancer.

In terms of balanced and complete nutritional content, spirulina and AFA can not compete with chlorella pyrenoidosa, but they still provide valuable nutritional supplement.

Vitamin B12 in spirulina is not assimilated by humans, as it is not a natural vitamin B12 but biologically inactive in humans as being a pseudo vitamin B12.

A COMPARISON BETWEEN CHLORELLA AND SPIRULINA

There are other edible algae such as spirulina, scenedesmus, chlorococcum, dunaliella salina and seaweeds which are used a lot by Oriental people.
But no other algae has such impressive properties as chlorella pyrenoidosa.
There are consumers who confuse chlorella and spirulina. Since the dried form of spirulina is also green, it is often difficult to distinguish the two algae.
Increased confusion may be due to the fact that both varieties are in tablet form, but although spirulina is an interesting algae, it cannot replace chlorella.
Spirulina is a multicellular spiral algae (bacteria), completely different from the single-celled round shape of chlorella (plant).
Although spirulina and chlorella look the same in tablet form, they differ scientifically altogether.
They belong entirely to different systems and different classes and orders.
Chlorella belongs to the class of chlorophycae and clorococale orders, while spirulina belongs to the class cyanophyceae (cyanobacteria) and nostocales order. Chlorella is, as previously mentioned, a single-celled plant, spirulina is a multicellular cyanobacteria.

Chlorella has a "true", fully identifiable nucleotide (nucleus) and measures about three to eight microns in size, while Spirulina is 100 times bigger than chlorella and lacks "genuine" nucleotides.

The main pigmenting in photosynthesis also separates the two algae. Chlorella produces chlorophyll a, b, and beta-carotene, while spirulina produces chlorophyll a, b, beta-carotene and phycocyanin.

They also differ structurally, because spirulina, in comparison, has neither chloroplasts nor cell membranes. Chlorella contains 5-10 times more chlorophyll (up to 7%) and 3 times more calcium than spirulina. Chlorella contains vitamin C, spirulina contains no vitamin C.

ONLY CHLORELLA IS CONTAINING CGF (chlorella growth factor)

What also separates chlorella pyrenoidosa significantly from many other algae, is the great scientific interest. Chlorella has been investigated by, inter alia, Rockefeller Foundation, Carnegie Institute, Pasteur Institute and NASA.

Chlorella has existed for a long time and still is interesting for medical research in countries such as the United States, Japan, Germany, Russia, France and Israel. Spirulina does not have the cell wall structure that chlorella has, which has proven so valuable because it can attract heavy metals and other toxins and expel them from the body through the intestinal tract.

It is this special cell construction and content that is combined with the unique and beneficial growth factor (CGF) that places chlorella pyrenoidosa at the front of all other algae.

It is worth noting the difference between chlorella pyrenoidosa and chlorella vulgaris (another plant-member of the chlorella family).

Chlorella pyrenoidosa is alone in containing important sporopollenin, a unique carotene-like polymer that has been identified as the substance that binds and re-moves hydrocarbon poisons such as DDT and PCB and the heavy metals mercury, cadmium and others.

THE CHLORELLA HISTORY
Scientists claim that, at the earliest stages of the earth's existence, the atmosphere consisted of lethal gases, carbon dioxide, methane and ammonia.
It is a possibility that green plants such as chlorella had the task of transforming this impossible mixture for us into an atmosphere in which both animals, plants and humans could live. It has been considered whether chlorella may be the first link in the food chain with a clearly defined cell nucleus within its cell wall.
If this is correct, chlorella, as one of the first green plants, would prove to be the origin of all of us today known plants.
Although chlorella has existed since the creation of the earth, it was first discovered the year 1890.

A Dutch microbiologist, M.W Beijerinck found it and performed the cultivation of Chlorella vulgaris in 1890. He discovered, that this edible algae he found in the sea by the Dutch coast that same year, had an im-portant content of protein and other nutrients why it appeared to be the most interesting subject to explore.
Mr. Beijerinck gave chlorella its name from the Latin word chloros, which indicates greenish and ella, which

means small. Later, chlorella has been found in fossils dating over 2,5 million years ago (Precambrian time).

In 1917, German biologist Lindner had the idea of using chlorella as nutritious feed with its content of more than 50% protein because at that time, there was a great famine going on in Germany. However, he finished his ongoing work at the end of World War I (1914-1918).

In 1931, German biochemist Heinrich Warburg received the Nobel Prize in Physiology or Medicine for his studies of photosynthesis in chlorella.

Another researcher by the name of Hardner, approached where Lindner stopped, but it was only the year 1948, as a third scientist named Kuick would finish and complete the first and fundamental research of chlorella's importance.
Lindner's, Hardner's and Kuick's researches were followed by other researchers in the United States in the late 1940s.
Dhyana Bewicke and Beverly A. Potter wrote, that during the 1940s, two researchers, Jorgensen and Convit, gave a soup made of concentrated chlorella to 80 patients at a leprosy treatment centre in Venezuela.
The improved health of these patients resulted in the the first evidence that micro algae could provide an extremely beneficial supplement.
    To investigate the possibility of using chlorella as a food in many countries where famine existed after the second world war, 1948, a pilot study was carried out at Stanford Research Institute USA. In this study, it

was found that chlorella easily could be cultivated continuously and that this algae had an unusually fast growth rate. Continuous studies were suspended temporarily as there was insufficient funding.

During the 1950s, the Carnegie Institute, USA, launched a study of chlorella under the direction of a known research organization named Arthur D. Little Inc.

A pilot plant was built where it was found that chlorella could be grown on a commercial basis and the researchers concluded that chlorella could become valuable as a solution to the extensive famine in the world.

The postwar era faced a very serious problem in terms of food shortages in Japan and in other countries.

The Japanese became pioneers seeking to develop a technology for the treatment and commercial production of chlorella.

In the Orient, where kelp had long been used and considered to be a good food, the interest in chlorella woke up when Dr. Hiroshi Tamiya from Japan, began experiments at the Tokugawa Biological Institute in 1951. Dr Tamiya's studies were supported by Rockefeller Foundation, USA and by the Japanese State, and along with other Japanese researchers, he developed the technology and processes of growing and cultivating chlorella on a large scale.

At the beginning of the 1950s, a process was eventually made to make chlorella's cell more suitable for human and animals by making it more easily digestible for more efficient absorption of its nutritional properties.

In 1957 an ideal organization formed the Japan Chlorella Research Centre, after which, the world's largest cultivation basin was constructed. State aid was subsequently formed by another organization called the Japan Chlorella Association.
The purpose was to seek commercialization of chlorella as food.
However, plans were stopped after two years due to the fact that other foods such as rice and wheat had become more accessible and that chlorella could not compete because of its higher price.
    One reason why chlorella could not be commercialized at this time, was its lower degree of digestion due to the strong cell wall.
Although the naturally strong cellular wall of chlorella had protected its nutrition in the cell for more than 2.5 billion years, it did not prove to be beneficial to humans until later.

In 1961   Dr. Melvin Calvin at the University of California won the Nobel Prize in Chemistry for his research on the pathway of carbon dioxide and assimilation in plants. Dr. Calvin used Chlorella in his research.

The digestive problem was resolved only in 1975 when a patented procedure was developed whereby chlorella's cell wall could be broken down to the extent that made it available for humankind to about 80%.
As this opportunity became known, the universities and scientists in the government's service joined the research of chlorella even in other countries such as in Germany, Russia, England, Israel and the China Republic.

Chlorella created by sun and water

Chlorella is cultivated in filtered fresh water pools.
Much of sunlight and clean and fresh water are necessary ingredients to grow and harvest the finest chlorella of the finest quality.

The algae are grown in special freshwater pools in the Far East such as China, Japan and Taiwan, where there are more than 320 sunny days per year.

Under good conditions with plenty of sunshine, clean water and clean air, chlorella can achieve a remarkable growth rate.

It can multiply 4 times during 20 -24 hours. A chlorella cell divides into four cells in this short period of time.

Chlorella pyrenoidosa of high quality, is not subjected to any form of bad processing and remains natural, 100% clean and totally impervious to attacks of insecticides, pesticides or other synthetic additives.

Because it is subjected to such large amounts of sunlight, the content of chlorophyll in chlorella is larger than in most plants on Earth.

Thanks to this wealth of chlorophyll, chlorella promotes the combustion of other substances like protein and also prevents the growth of harmful bacteria.

Not until 1977, when they found a way to make it more digestible and thereby nutritionally more accessible to the body, people began to commercially use Chlorella as healthy food, not only In Japan, but also in the United States.

Especially in Japan, with an annual production of more than 2000 ton, chlorella is now considered to be the most important functional food on the market.

Chlorella is today registered as "Functional Food No.1" in Japan, where more than thirty million people are eating it every day.

In the 1960s, people investigated the possibility of using chlorella to produce oxygen and food for expeditions into outer space.
A kind of "algae space race" developed therefore between USA and Russia.

Space Program within NASA, US and space scientists institutions in the Soviet Union, have long tested and applied chlorella in space flights, as it is both a nutritious food and useful in connection with acquiring an efficient switching system for oxygen/carbon dioxide.

Dr. Oswald showed that the algae could support a grown man's entire metabolism. Mr. Kondratyev, as well as other space scientists in Russia, copied the information and found chlorella to be an ideal food when traveling in outer space.

What really is interesting to researchers around the world, is chlorella's growth ability, which hardly has its equal.

Chlorella can continually be harvested under controlled conditions and its growth has a capacity of an estimated 40-50 tons per acre and year, compared with rice as with abundant irrigation, can achieve a growth rate of 2 tons per acre and year.

Chlorella is grown in freshwater basins in countries with numerous sunny days as in Taiwan, where it originally started to be grown on a large scale followed by industrial growth in both Japan and the United States.

In these basins the water is kept in motion for 24 hours a day, year around.

It is also the cultivation of chlorella, which is subjected to constant surveillance included rigorous hygiene controls and frequent analysis.

In laboratories, the chlorella cells of the highest qualities are sorted out first, after which these are collected in bottles before being transferred to small cultivation ponds.

When the density reaches to the next step, chlorella is moved to large well-guarded cultivation ponds for their cleanliness and further hygienic treatment.

When chlorella is ready to be harvested, it is moved to a special tank and then to an ultracentrifugation machine where it is washed and centrifuged with high pressure to separate cells wherein it also is dried to some degree.

From here chlorella is air dried in quite low heat for a few seconds.

Throughout the whole production process, chlorella cells are controlled and analyzed for hygiene and nutritional content that are the most important key issues.

Chlorella powder could then be cold pressed into tablets, using its own fiber content, which means that no binders or other tablet devices are added.

Although the algae grow naturally in fresh water, chlorella destined for human consumption is generally cultivated outdoors in mineral rich freshwater ponds under direct sunlight. The entire process from strain maintenance in the laboratory to harvesting of the final product is monitored by microbiologists to ensure optimal nutrient value and product purity.

It should be noted that all cultivations and processing of chlorella are not always of good quality.

It is therefore important to, in the first place, inform yourselves of the chlorella you want to use and that it is of the highest quality and therefore should be pro-duced and processed under the strictest quality standards.

Chlorella is one of the main export products in Taiwan and Japan, where the most famous plantations work under very strict quality conditions.

Comparing to other algae, Chlorella is superior in several respects.
The chloroplasts in chlorella are adapted to rapid photosynthesis that made it grow faster than most other plants. Chlorella has a higher percentage of protein and nucleic material. All cell functions are controlled from the nucleus.
Chlorella can increase the growth rate of lactobacillus that is a combination between sulphur nucleotide with protein and nucleic acid. This is due to the Chlorella Growth Factor (CGF).

Chlorella is used all over the world by health professionals to help remove heavy metals such as mercury and cadmium from the bodies of patients showing signs of heavy metal toxicity.

In Japan, the chlorella facts are so convincing that the algae are popularly consumed in whole food supplement form because of the country's history of exposure to nuclear radiation.
Also of all the wide variety of protocols available to safely removing of mercury amalgam fillings, the majority of them include the consumption of chlorella before and after removal.

Chlorophyll literally soaks up residual mercury in your body and it then eliminates it through your lymph system (by sweating) and also through your bowels.

Chlorella can help to treat cardiovascular ailments (lowering cholesterol and triglycerides), liver conditions, kidney conditions, diabetes, hypertension, wound healing, fighting anaemia by stimulating production of red blood cells, arthritis, digestive conditions, tissue detoxification (including detoxification of heavy metals), skin problems and strengthening of the immune function.

It can also stimulate healing in the body and promotes growth in young individuals and allows repair to damaged tissues in mature individuals. It can also help to deodorize and freshen the breath.

If you are consuming a lot of mercury contaminated sea fish, it is advisable to also consume chlorella pyrenoidosa.

Due to its extraordinary ability to bind with toxic metals, chlorella pyrenoidosa from Taiwan, cultivated in sunlight and in a cleaner climate than any other country that produces chlorella, can be of great importance to all people in the world.

The chlorophyll in chlorella benefits and cleanses the liver that is the chief organ for detoxing our body on a daily basis. If your liver is functioning at its optimal level, it will speed up the process of detoxification from the myriad of poisons we come in contact with on a regular basis every day.

The chlorella facts have shown this. Even if you eat all organic food and live far away from any major cities, you are still exposed to a wide variety of environmental toxins.

Chlorella is considered to be a first class detoxifying agent, capable of removing alcohol from the liver, heavy metals such as cadmium and mercury, certain pesticides, herbicides, and poly-chlorinated biphenyls (PCBs) from the body's tissues.

Chlorella can also absorb toxins from the intestines, relieving chronic constipation, alter bacterial contents in the bowel and eliminate intestinal gas. It is also effective in healing skin wounds both mild and severe.

From a nutritional perspective, chlorella is a perfect food. The whole food is eaten because each chlorella cell is a complete plant with all of its attributes intact.

Added to this fact it is 100% natural, pure, and not poisoned by chemical additives or pesticide residues as it is cultured in pure, clean water with nutrient input. It remains unspoiled for years and it has only 400-600 calories per 100 grams.

In fact, chlorella algae contain so much food subtances, that forty years ago, both the World Bank and the United Nations declared it to be the healthiest food in the world.

Even NASA says, "one gram of chlorella has the nutritional equivalent of 1,000 grams of fruits and vegetables!

German biochemist and cell physiologist Otto Heinrich Warburg, who was awarded with the Nobel Prize in Physiology or Medicine in 1931 for his research on cell respiration also studied the photosynthesis of Chlorella.

There are over 12 genetically different varieties of chlorella. The best known representatives of the species, are chlorella **pyrenoidosa** and chlorella **vulgaris.**

In spite of their genetically resemblance, **Chlorella pyrenoidosa** possesses particular characteristics which makes it an exceptional food or as a food supplement also within the medical faculty.

Some growers of chlorella says that they are fermenting their algae in tanks and that the plant is as healthy as chlorella grown in direct sunlight.
But it could not be the truth, as high quality of chlorella has been growing in direct sunlight for as long as there has been plant life on Earth. And we must not forget the richness of nutrients that is coming through the sunlight.
There is only fungus like certain mushrooms that grows without sunlight and they do not produce chlorophyll.

It is the effects of the **pyrenoidosa** (sorokiniana) variety, cultivated in direct sunlight that is to be described in this book.
Chlorella is known to be a powerful aid to the body remediation of heavy metals and other pesticides.
Detoxification means removal of toxic substances from the body.
This is a natural process that the body must constantly undergo when we are daily exposed to exogenous toxic substances, pesticides, pharmaceuticals, heavy metals or toxins produced in the body such as in the intestine by inefficient metabolism.
Many people believe that Chlorella can serve as a potential source of food and energy because its photosynthetic efficiency can, in theory, reach 8% comparable with other highly efficient crops such as sugar cane.

Today, chlorella is used by people all around the world and is looked upon as a great super food, helping to inhibit and treat problems of different kinds.
This little green micro-algae have ancient ancestry (pre-Cambrian time, over 3,5 billion years ago) but

was first discovered by the microbiologist M.W. Beijerinck in 1890 when he found chlorella off the Dutch coast and could begin the research.

A Japanese dioxin study provides convincing evidence that one of the easiest ways to protect you from the harmful effects of persistent organized pollutants (Pops), is to consume a high-quality chlorella pyrenoidosa supplement every day.

Chlorella contains digestives and other enzymes. They are enzymes such as **chlorophyllaese** and **pepsin** (digestive) enzymes that perform a lot of body functions.

Chlorella has many different types of enzymes, which our bodies are in need of.

Clinical trials suggested that daily dietary supplementation with Chlorella may reduce high blood pressure, lower serum cholesterol, accelerate wound healing, and enhance immune functions.

Its possibility to relieve symptoms, improve quality of life and normalize body functions in patients suffering from the illnesses studied here, suggests that larger and more comprehensive clinical trials of chlorella are warranted for these as well as other chronic illnesses.

A closer look at chlorella.

Chlorella is a single cellular green micro algae (2-8 microns in diameter) and has a true nucleus.

Chlorella is grown in freshwater basins and is considered by the scientific expertise in medical research around the world, to be the most interesting and nutritional, edible algae. Chlorella cells are round in shape and its size can be compared to human blood cells. Chlorella pyrenoidosa has been able to maintain its pure genetic structure for over 3.5 billion years, which has been verified by scientific studies of fossils from the Pre-Cambrian times. The discovery shows that this is possible when chlorella's nutritional content is protected by its strong cell wall. The cell wall contains the following substances:

27% protein	9,2% fat
15,4% alpha cellulose	31 % hemicellulose
3,3 % glucosamine	5,2 % iron and calcium

Chlorella belongs to the group of green micro algae. There are 15 members of the chlorella family, of which both Chlorella pyrenoidosa and Chlorella vulgaris are considered to be the most interesting from a nutritional point of view.

These are relatively similar to each other, but Chlorella pyrenoidosa is considered to be the most interesting of the two, thanks to its more complete and balanced nutritional content.
Chlorella pyrenoidosa is also the one of the two that contains the important *sporopollenin*, a polymeric substance capable of attracting heavy metals and bringing these toxins through the intestinal tract.

Unlike multicellular plants, chlorella is a single cell algae which also means that each cell is a self-sufficient organism.
Each cell has its own organs and functions to live alone. A 3 micron-small chlorella cell grows with help of the sun's energy and carbon dioxide in fresh water during the process of photosynthesis.

Chlorella pyrenoidosa contains 50-70% protein based on 19 amino acids.
With a reproduction that is about fifty times faster than other protein sources, this small algae can be an important source of protein in developing countries as well as in countries where the population is too large in relation to their cultivation capacity.

Chlorella pyrenoidosa also contains other necessary nutrients. In addition to being composed of the largest amount of chlorophyll of all the seedling on Earth, this algae is also rich in vitamins, minerals, fibers, nucleic acids, DNA/RNA, amino acids, enzymes, fatty acids and Chlorella Growth Factor (CGF).

The Chlorella cell is hardly visibly to the human eye.
Chlorella's rapid growth is completely unmatched by its quadrupling of 20-25 hours under favorable conditions like a lot of sunshine, clean water and clean air.

If chlorella had the possibility to reproduce itself freely, it could have generated very rapidly itself to the equivalent of earth's surface. However, the growth rate is limited by the fact that a chlorella cell requires a lot of sun and if an abundance of chlorella would cause a lack of available cultivation space to be able to repro-duce itself, the growth would decrease.

Thanks to chlorella's rapid growth, the microscopic algae has attracted great scientific interest around the world.

The algae has been examined as well-balanced nu-trition for the future as the population on the earth increases so rapidly that it poses a high risk of future extensive nutritional deficiencies.

Chlorella's cell wall consists of three layers of which the thicker in the centre contains cellulose fibre (sporopollenin).

Atkinson and employees found that the chlorella cell wall consists of 14 nm thick, three lamellae layers that proved to be extremely resistant and considered to consist of a polymerized carotene-like material.
Chlorella's cell wall is 27% proteins, 9.2% lipids, 15.4% alpha cellulose, 31% hemicellulose, 3.3% glucose and 5.2% ashes (containing iron and calcium).

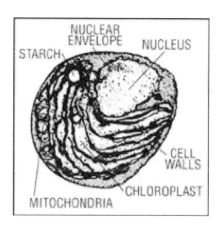

This chlorella cell looks small and simple though it is very rich and a complete individual with a well defined structure.

The nucleus (N) is contained in the nuclear envelope (NE), outside of which are the chloroplast (C) and mitochondria (M), with a grain of starch (S) off in the "northwest" quadrant: the cell walls confine and defend the whole unit.

If we look at a chlorella cell in cross section, using an electron microscope with 31200 times magnification, we see a cell wall that protects the cell from contamination and degradation. The chlorella cell is approximately as small as a human blood cell (0.002-0.008 mm) and is the first form of a cell with a clearly defined nucleotide (nucleus).

The cell has a convex-like chloroplast that contains chlorophyll and a core and mitochondrial where nutrition turns into energy and starch.

The core is surrounded by a double casing with openings, which we call core pores. These are the centers of amino acids.

Chlorella's cell wall protects the cell nucleus and its nutritional content until growing and cultivation of the algae is completed.

In order to make it more digestible (76-80%) for human and animals, special processes are used, for example the Dyno-Mill method or Ultra Air Drying System, which means that the algae can still maintain its full nutritional value.

There are other systems for the degradation of chlorella's cell wall in order to make it more easy to digest, but it is recommended that you use only chlorella treated with recognized methods.

There are the the properties of chlorella's cell wall that make this alga so unique. It promotes the body's attempts to relieve itself from hydrocarbons and heavy metals such as lead, cadmium, uranium, mercury and other foreign substances such as DDT and PCB. In chlorella's cell wall there is an active substance called **sporopollin**.

This particular substance found only in **Chlorella pyrenoidosa** has the ability to bind to different heavy metals and maintain them.

Subsequently, cell wall fractions emit these toxins from the body through the intestinal tract.

After studying a large amount of scientific literature on chlorella, researchers seem to have come to the conclusion that it is mainly four main components that have been identified as responsible for special health effects.

These are chlorophyll, the unique cell wall, vitamin A, beta carotene, and the CGF (chlorella growth factor).

Chlorella, by the way, has a variety of properties that are helpful for organs and tissues that have been injured for various reasons.

Science believes that chlorella can help normalize too high or too low values, which means it stimulates balancing of the body's different functions. Chlorella's ultra-fast growth and propagation ability is due to its nuclear (core) distinctive features.

This is the reason for the discovery, that this algae has abilities to stimulate cell repair in human and animals, as well as to stimulate the faster recovery of a number of known diseases.

Chlorella is very rich in chlorophyll, the richest source of protein among all known plants on earth, which, along with the special cell wall of the algae, helps to purify blood, kidneys, liver, air organs, and to feed the intestinal flora and thereby strengthen the effect of being so necessary cellulose lactobacilli. In addition, fragments of the cell wall (cellulose) absorb heavy metals such as cadmium, lead, PCB, uranium and mercury contained in the body and effectively transport these toxins through the intestinal tract.

Chlorella is rich in nucleic acids DNA/RNA. It contains vitamins A, B1, B2, B6, B12, C, D, E K, niacin, pantothenic acid, folic acid, PABA, inositol and minerals such as calcium, magnesium, iron, zinc, copper, phosphorus, iodine, cobalt, manganese and traces of sulfur and selenium. Chlorella is also rich in fatty acids, including omega-3 and omega-6, and consists of more than 60% protein in the form of 19 amino acids, including all 8 essentials that are necessary. Chlorella's protein quality and composition of amino acids can be compared to animated proteins, with the exception of less content of methionine.

However, and in some cases when it comes to cancer, it can be an advantage as a number of cases of cancer tumors are dependent on methionine for its growth. Protein in chlorella is superior to animal protein such as in meat and eggs.

The body must first break down meat and egg to its composition of amino acids before it can use them for its individual protein need.

Chlorella is a complete diet that provides us with nutrition at the cellular level.

Scientists claim that single-celled algae make up the first link in the food chain, making all life possible on earth, and algae is the first form of life developed on our planet.

Single cellular protein sources are rich in nucleic acids due to their concentration of RNA and DNA. Fats rich in nucleic acids transmit cell-protective effects, which can help us achieve a long, healthy life. The body can immediately absorb and use components of nucleic acids, which saves on energy that would otherwise have to be used to synthesize them. What we find in chlorella's biochemical makeup is an amount of nutrition that is very similar to the nutrition necessary for the human cell. Chlorella provides us with complete, well-balanced and essential nutrition.

The most important thing in this context is however, that our body genetically recognizes this nutrition, and thus can easily utilize and use it efficiently.

In addition to being a rich source of protein, chlorella also supplies us with carbohydrates, essential fatty acids, minerals, vitamins, chlorophyll, fibers, antioxidants, RNA and DNA, chlorella growth factor (CGF) and an amount of phyto-chemicals.

Nutrients in chlorella pyrenoidosa fully fill the body's requirements to be considered a superior healthy functional food.

Chlorella promotes and nourishes and stimulates each of the over 75 trillion cells that we have in our body.

Because cells are fundamental building blocks in the body's different parts, the minimum limitation on their natural activities can lead to degradation effects.

Chlorella can provide the body with important nutritional support, which is usually lacking in the daily food and life of the industrial society.

It represents an ideal nutritional supplement for the whole family, from toddlers to adult children, adults and seniors. **Especially important it is to eat Chlorella pyrenoidosa before, during and after a pregnancy. Chlorella's nutritional support is excellent for people suffering from a lifelong debilitating disease, or with a broken or weakened body system.**

Refined and processed foods, treated for our convenience, have simultaneously depleted our soil. Whole grains, legumes, fruits and vegetables have been replaced by nutritious carbohydrates such as refined flour and sugar. With today's soiled soil, farming methods, transplantation and long shipment and storage times, "healthy" natural food lacks some of the key vitamins and minerals that are so vital to us and our immune system.

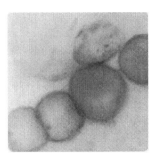

Fossils of chlorella

Chlorella and chlorophyll
Chlorella has got its name due to its significant content of chlorophyll. Chlorella contains 2%-7% chlorophyll per gram.
Chlorophyll is one of the most important nutrients that contribute to more effective cleansing of intestines and other liver and blood elimination systems. Green algae are the most prominent source of chlorophyll in the plant world, and of all plants, Chlorella pyrenoidosa has the largest content of chlorophyll.
Chlorella contains up to five times more chlorophyll than wheat grass, more than four times more than

Spirulina, over 12 times more than grain and about 50 times more than alfalfa.

It was only during the two centuries that humans began to understand how fundamental it is with green plants for all life on our planet and how vital it is with chlorophyll for all vegetation. Somehow, the Greek philosophers, being considered to have been the first scientists were right when they claimed that chloro-phyll captures the power of the sun and uses it to give life to our plants. Chlorophyll is the green pigment of plants that enables photosynthesis.

During synthesis, the cells absorb carbon dioxide from the environment and release oxygen.

This means that chlorophyll helps cells to capture and convert all sunlight into energy and, on the other hand, make the plants green; the word chlorophyll comes from Greek chloros = green, phyllum = leaf.

All living on earth derives directly or indirectly from the sunlight falling on the chlorophyll.

Phytoplankton is a collective name for all photo-synthetic microorganisms in the seas, the most im-portant of which are green algae and cyanobacteria.

It is estimated that these count for at least half of the photosynthesis on earth. One can say that they conse-quently have a decisive effect on the global climate.

Through the absorption of carbon dioxide which is the most important of the greenhouse gases, the green-house effect is moderated. It was only during the sixteenth century, when the microscope was invented, as scientists began to get some clarity in the mystery of plants' lives.

It was found that there were more interesting details around the plant than could be seen with the eyes. Likewise, with the help of the microscope, a liquid was found that floated in the veins of the leaves, as well as tests on small holes or pores through which the plants seemed to breathe.

In 1772, a British chemist, Joseph Priestley, came under the process of photosynthesis. In the daylight, Priestley saw green leaves that "inhaled" carbon dioxide through their blood pores, mixed it with water to make carbohydrates and exhaled a mysterious gas that allowed iron to rust and the flame of light to flare up.
The year 1774 Priestley named this gas, oxide (oxygen).
It was discovered that the leaflets' cells contained smaller "sub-cells" called chloroplasts in which the process of photosynthesis occurred.
Each chloroplast contained thousands of green pigment granules called chlorophyll.
Somehow, these chlorophyll grains caught the vitality of solar energy, used it to share water molecules and reunite them with carbon dioxide to make plant sugar (carbohydrates).
This plant sugar was used to build cellulose, the structural material in plant growth and all other substances necessary for the plant. All leftover plant sugar is stored either in roots or in the fruit itself.
The chloroplasts in the plant cell have their own DNA, make their own protein and reproduce themselves.
They are not made by the cells. As the algae cells are divided, the chloroplasts are divided into the algae.

Dr. Richard Willstatter received the Nobel Prize in 1915 for his discovery of the chlorophyll's chemical structure, a network of carbon, nitrogen, hydrogen and oxygen atoms surrounding a single magnesium atom. 15 years later, Dr. Hans Fisher received the Nobel Prize for his work on clarifying the chemical structure of hemoglobin. To his surprise, he found that hemoglobin, to a large extent, resembled chlorophyll.

Chlorophyll is simply the blood of the plants.
Hemoglobin is the color pigment that gives the blood cells its red color, chlorophyll is the pigment that gives the plants its green color.
When Dr. Fisher separated the color pigment from the protein molecule, it showed that the biggest difference between blood and chlorophyll was that, the former has an iron atom in its center while the chlorophyll center has a magnesium atom. Differences and similarities in our blood and chlorophyll are very interesting. Both are pigments that perform their functions in cells and both are vital to the organism to which they belong. Both work with carbon dioxide and oxygen and both are similar in structure.

Among the differences, blood has iron in its center, chlorophyll has magnesium in its centre; blood absorbs oxygen and releases carbon dioxide while chlorophyll absorbs carbon dioxide and emits oxygen, blood is red, chlorophyll is green.

After having found the similarity between blood and chlorophyll, Dr. Fisher, along with many other scientists and researchers in America, started studies of chlorophyll for medical use.

To name some of the extensive medical tests done with chlorophyll, doctors at Temple University, USA, used chlorophyll in-packs, ointments and solutions to treat 1200 patients whose symptoms covered everything from broken appendicitis with spread infections to common cold. Chlorophyll mixed with sterilized water was used to wash clean deep, in many cases, highly infected wounds after surgery. Wound healing, spinal cord, bone marrow inflammation and superficial open wounds were purified with a solution of chlorophyll or covered with chlorophyll salve.

The researchers found in test tubes that chlorophyll was not directly healing, but on the other hand, it was discovered that it increased the resilience of the cells and thus prevented the growth of the bacteria. Between 1947 and 1951, 1755 patients were tested at Loyola University College of Dentistry (with 618 controls).

It was found that using chlorophyll in toothpaste, you could check or stop the symptoms of gingivitis (inflammation of the gum), simple dental infection and mouth ulcers.

The head of the research team, Dr Gustav Rapp, claimed that chlorophyll can reduce bacteria associated with tooth decay up to 8 hours, while other common antiseptics did not achieve any improvement. Other specialists have also reported very positive results when using chlorophyll.

Dr. Burgi and his co-workers used chlorophyll in patients with anemia, tuberculosis, heart disease, atherosclerosis and depression. The latter through its enhancing effect (tonic). Haven FL, J Biol. Chem., 118: 111-1221

Over 1000 cases of respiratory infections, sinusitis and other colds were treated and showing very good results under the supervision of Dr. Robert Ridpath and Dr. T Carroll Davis.
Chlorophyll is also considered to be the primary natural cleansing agent for tissues, not only by it's control of calcium in the body, but also because it cleans liver and gallbladder.

Some of the chlorophyll's beneficial effects.
Protects stomach walls, inhibiting pepsin activities
Anti-mutagenic: against aflatoxin B (toxin)
Anti-Oxidant
Deodorizing (body odor, bad breath and others).
Excretes toxic dioxin
Provides iron, builds red blood count and improves anemia conditions.
Cleans and deodorizes bowel tissues
Purifies the liver and aids agains hepatitis.
Feeds iron to heart tissues.
Heels sores, soothes inflamed tonsils, ulcers and painful hemorrhoids and piles.
Feeds heart tissues and improves varicose.
Regulates menstruation and improve production of milk.
Aids hemophilia, improves diabetes and asthma.
Resist bacteria in wounds.
Cleans tooth and gum structure.
Relieves sore throat
Soothes sore ulcer tissues

Chlorophyll also helps to digest heavy proteins and fats, facilitate the absorption of iron, clean and dilate the blood, as well as provide fiber with a view to healing the intestinal tract. Experiments within the US Army have shown that chlorella, as being rich in chlorophyll, can effectively influence the negative effects of radioactive radiation.

Dr. Bernard Jensen explains that chlorophyll can be used as antidote to pesticides and can help eliminate poisons from the body.

Chlorophyll is a powerful cleanser and a good stimulus for the production of hemoglobin in the blood. It helps to remove toxic material from our internal organs and thus allow the onset of a natural healing process. Chlorophyll also benefits healthy people because its activities strengthen the resistance to all sorts of diseases. As an addition, inflammatory conditions such as arthritis and gastric ulcer respond well to the intake of green algae according to Paul Pitchford, author of Healing with Whole Foods.

Chlorophyll can also help reduce cell damage caused by environmental carcinogens by acting as an antioxidant, the chemist Karl J. Abrams writes in his book, *Algae to the Rescue (Logan House)*. P

Pitchford and others state the theory that chlorophyll resembles the human blood cell. "The ability of chlorophyll to enrich blood deficiency can depend on a similarity in the molecular structure between hemoglobin (red blood cells) and chlorophyll," he writes. "Their molecules are virtually identical to the exception of respective center (atom): The center of the chlorophyll molecule is magnesium, while iron occupies the central site of the hemoglobin."

Hemoglobin is an oxygen-carrying, iron-rich protein in the red blood cells (erythrocytes) that transport oxygen and give the blood its red color.

Chlorophyll is also effective in anemia and stimulates the production of red blood cells in the body.

A number of researchers have proposed the use of chlorophyll as medical therapy for anemia.

Chlorophyll helps to acidify the body and also the brain. Chlorella is sometimes referred to as "Brain Food". Chlorella has the highest concentration of chlorophyll that exists, from 1.7% to 7.0% and in addition, this greenhouse is a whole vegetable food, whose content consists of many other protective, health-promoting vitamins and minerals. Chlorella gives us large amounts of chlorophyll without the need to use chemically produced products. It can be mentioned that a single tablet corresponds to about 35 tablets made of alfalfa, which is taken quite often as a chlorophyll supplement.

CULTIVATING CHLORELLA *PYRENOIDOSA*.
STEP 1

Chlorella pyrenoidosa cells that have to respond to the desired physical characters are investigated and collected under the microscope and placed in breeding cylinders of glass containing nutrient solution.

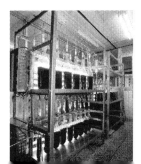
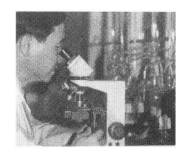

After the first reproductive stage of Chlorella, where it has reached a particular maturity, it is moved to a larger glass container to continue the reproductive process. Temperature and humidity in the cultivation area must be serviced and maintained at optimal levels throughout the process.

STEP 2
When the cultivation of chlorella reaches the required maturity in reproductive containers, it is moved to an outdoor enclosure for accelerating its growth under natural conditions.
Cultivation is now sufficiently strong to be able to adapt and thrive in the outdoor environment.
The water in the cultivation basins is in constant motion by a mechanical mixing ramp.

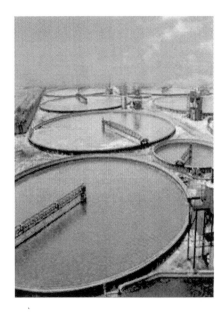

Outdoor Cultivation

This ensures and provides a guarantee, that the chlorella cells get similar and sufficient amount of sunlight, nutrients and carbon dioxide, which is essential to the process of photosynthesis to go right. Chlorella remains in the outdoor pool until it is ready to be harvested.
The time for the process vary throughout the year but ranges from 7 days in summer period to about 10 days in wintertime.

STEP 3
When chlorella is ready for harvest, the algae-rich water is moved through a pipeline to a tank where it is filtered to be separated from the excess water and any other particles. The algae are repeatedly washed during a constant supply of fresh water.
Centrifugal force separates the algae from the water, which is removed and leaving a crop of pure chlorella.

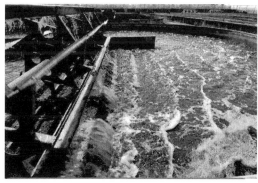 Harvest and wash

After harvesting concentrated and cleaned, Chlorella pyrenoidosa (sorokiniana) solution is pumped into a Spray Dryer and when spraying it the pressure drops from high to low pressure instantly and the solution is being sprayed out.

Chlorella is then dried through an air-drying system, which transforms the wet algae concentrate to clean and fine powder.
At this moment, the cell wall is partially cracked due to this drastically change in pressure.
With the hot air inside the spray dryer (temperature is around 150-160 degrees C), the Chlorella is dried very quickly.

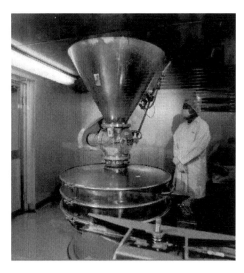

Drying

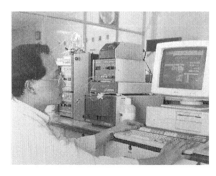

Quality control

STEP 4
Quality control is essential and is carried throughout the cultivation and harvesting process. Samples are taken from each harvest, mixed with brine (Brine is a solution of salt (usually sodium chloride) in water.

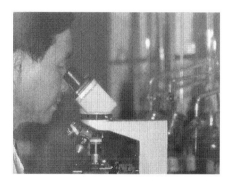

In different contexts, brine may refer to salt solutions ranging from about 3.5%, a typical concentration of seawater, or the lower end of solutions used for brining foods).
It is a culture prepared to carefully examine if there is a presence of bacteria.
Subsequently the computer system is controlling chlorella's nutritional content and if not fully of satisfactory in accordance with established standards (food grade), it is processed for sale as an ingredient for animal feed.

Completion.
After the chlorophyll content has been measured and approved of, using a color spectra-photometer, the examination of the algae finally is finished under the microscope in order to be able to ensure its cleanliness before the product is then to be packaged.

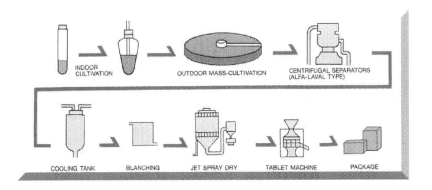

Chlorella must abide by the strict rules of good standard in order to be sold for human consumption.

General analysis (per 100 g)

Moisture	5,3 %
Crude protein	3,3 %
Crude fat	38,5 %
Carbohydrate	2,6 %
Crude fibre	0,2 %
Dietary fiber	8,60%
Crude ash	68,1 %
Calories	426 cal
Sodium	43 mg
Lutein	149,6 ppm

10 % RNA
3 % DNA

Fatty acids per 100 gr.

Unsaturated	81,8 %
Saturated	28,5 %
Chlorophyll	2608 mg
Xanthophyll	155.0 mg

Vitamins (100 g)

Vitamin A activity	55.500.0 IU
Alpha-Carotene	24.0 mg
Beta-Carotene	1.11 mg
Thiamin (B1)	1.66 mg
Riboflavin (B2)	5.4 mg
Niacin (B3)	25.0 mg
Biotin (B7)	191.6 mcg
Pantothenic Acid (B5)	2.0 mg
Pyridoxin (B6)	2.97 mg
Cobalamin (B12)	40,29 ug
Folic Acid (B9)	17.0 mg
Pyrodaxal	0.58 mg
Pyridoxine	0,08 mg
Pyridoxamine	2,34 mg
PABA (B10)	0.60 mg
Vitamin C	49,8 mg
Calciferol (Vit D, int. Unit)	23000 IE
Vitamin E (a-Tocopherol)	17.48 mg
Phylloquinone (Vitamin K1)	2.2 mg
Inositol (I)	198 mg

Minerals (per 100 g)

Potassium	915,1 mg
Calcium	357,8 mg
Phosphorus	1324 mg
Magnesium	316,4 mg
Iron	62,2 mg

Zinc (Zn)	2,4 mg
Copper	0,08 mg
Sodium	43 mg
Iodine	0.10 mg
Manganese	171 ug
Cobalt	Trace of
Selenium	Trace of
Sulphur	Trace of

Amino Acids (per 100 g)

L-Arginine	3171,22 mg
L-Lysine.	4443.03 mg
L-Histidine*	1028.41 mg
L-Tyrosine	1888.73 mg
L-Leucine*	4411.10 mg
L-Isoleucine *	1799.80 mg
L-Methionine*	903.44 mg
L-Valine*	2882.33 mg
L-Alanine	4818.01 mg
Glycine	3052.77 mg
L(-)Proline	2749.71 mg
L-Glutamic Acid	6197.80 mg
L-Serine	1867.96 mg
L-Threonine*	2170.53 mg
L-Aspartic Acid	4482.80 mg
L-Tryptophan*	1090,00 mg
L(-)Cystine	286.18 mg
Total Nitrogen	10.96 g

*) Essential amino acids

a-Linoleic Acid (GLA) (omega 6)	2170 mg
a-Linolenic Acid (ALA) (omega 3)	3180 mg
C14:0 0.6 %	
C14:1 0.9 %	

C14:2   0.9 %
C16:0 15.6 %
C16:1   9.1 %
C16:2   5.5 %
C16:3 17.1 %
C18:0   2.0 %
C18:1 10.0 %
C18:2 15.5 %
C18:3 22.8 %

Chlorella contains all of the following:

- amino acids
- protein
- chlorophyll
- vitamins
- minerals
- beta-carotene
- dietary fiber
- antioxidants
- bioactive substances
- enzymes
- fiber
- lipids
- carbohydrates

Chlorella is about 60% protein and able to produce this protein 50 times more efficiently than other protein crops.

This is why chlorella is a perfect food and protein source for many people in the world. Chlorella contains all 8 essential amino acids, the constituents of protein.

Its amino acid is easily compared with that of animal derived protein, except that it has a lower amount of Methionine.

Chlorella contains more chlorophyll than any other plant on earth.

CARBOHYDRATES

Carbohydrates are vital for humans. They provide fuel to the body if you chose the right sort. Carbohydrates fuels are in bread, beans, milk, potatoes, spaghetti, coconut fat and wheat. Green plants as Chlorella is using the photosynthesis to combine carbon dioxide with water to make carbon hydrates.

Carbohydrates can be stored in the liver and muscles using insulin and cortisol (steroid hormone).

Carbs can be stored in the liver and Glucose is easily absorbed in the blood and delivered to the cells in all organs, glands, tissues and body systems and transforms into energy. The brain uses about 25% glucose or blood sugar.

Carbohydrates are broken down into single sugar by the enzymes activity. Most fruits and vegetables are classified as complex carbohydrates such as, for example potatoes.

The main benefit of these carbohydrates is that they provide a steady stream of sugar to the blood, which stabilizes energy production. Chlorella contains about 20% carbohydrates.

Space programs in NASA, USA and space scientists in the Soviet Union have long been testing and applying chlorella in space travels as nutritional food and in connection with obtaining an efficient oxygen/carbon dioxide exchange system. During the 1960s, the possibility of using chlorella was investigated to produce oxygen and food in the outer space.

A kind of algae space race was developed between the US and Russia. Oswald showed that the chlorella algae could support an adult's entire metabolism.

The result of this survey was soon copied by Kondratyev and other space researchers in Russia, where chlorella was found to be an ideal food when traveling in the outer space. What mostly interested other researchers around the world, is chlorella's growth ability, which is hardly contradictory. Chlorella can continuously be harvested under controlled conditions.

Growth has a capacity of estimated 40-50 tons per acre and year, compared with rice as, with heavy irrigation and fertilizer, grows 2 tonnes per acre and year. Chlorella is grown in freshwater basins in countries with lots of sun included. In Taiwan, where it originally began to grow on a large scale, followed by industrial cultivation in both Japan and the United States.

In these pools the water is in motion for 24 hours per day all year round. The cultivation of chlorella is also here subject to constant growth control including hygienic controls and analysis.

When chlorella is ready to be harvested, it is moved to a special tank and then to an ultra centrifugal machine where it is washed and centrifuged at high turns to separate cells, and it is also dried to some extent.

From here, chlorella is air-dried completely in low heat for a few seconds. During the entire production process, the product is checked and analyzed, as hygiene and nutritional content are the key issues.

Chlorella powder is then cold-pressed into tablets using its own fibre content, which means that no binders or other aids should be added.

It should be noted that all cultivation and treatment of chlorella does not always correspond to quality.

It is therefore important that you first know that the chlorella you want to use is of the highest quality and should therefore be manufactured and processed under strictest quality requirements.

Chlorella is one of the most important export products in Taiwan and Japan, where the most well known crops work under extremely strict quality conditions.

Thanks to chlorella's rapid growth, these microscopic algae have attracted great scientific interest around the world.

The algae have been examined as well-balanced nutrition in the future as population growth on earth increases so rapidly that it poses the risk of future extensive nutritional deficiencies.

Chlorella's Amino Acids and Proteins

Amino acids are the protein building blocks and unlike the other two basic nutrients, sugar and fatty acids, amino acids contain about 16% of nitrogen.

Due to the beneficial functions of the amino acids, it is very important to ensure that the body receives this nutrition, either in connection with the daily food or as a dietary supplement. Protein is needed for each living organism and next to water, protein is the largest proportion of body weight because it is found in muscles, organs, hair.

The protein used for the body's structure does not originate directly from the diet but is broken down into amino acids.

The body then transforms these, as needed to specific proteins. Amino acids are used in most of the body's processes from controlling the body's movements to the brain's functions.

One refers to about 25 amino acids in human health.

The liver produces about 80% of these amino acids, because the rest, 20% must be supplied through the diet, and then called the essential amino acids. These essential amino acids are histidine, isoleucine, leucine, lysine, methionine, phenylalanine, threonine, tryptophan and valine.

The other about 80% that can be manufactured by the liver, include alanine, arginine, asparagine, aspartic acid, cysteine, cystine, glutamic acid, glycine, ornithine, proline, serine, tyrosine and taurine.

The functions of the amino acids are interrelated and a balanced and healthy supply of this nutrition is necessary in order to establish and maintain good body functions.

Nutritional deficiencies in amino acids have a negative impact on our health just like other stressors such as trauma, drug use, aging, infections, daily stress etc.

When the body synthesizes protein, ammonia is formed as waste in the liver. When excessive intake of protein occurs through the diet, more ammonia is formed, which gives the liver even more work with the task of rinsing the waste.

Supplements of amino acids are available in different forms but can be divided in three types, either from animal, yeast or vegetable protein.

Most amino acids can be produced in two types with the exception of glycine, which are either in D-form or L-form.

Man prefers the L-form.

Chlorella pyrenoidosa is a very interesting source of protein, because the algae contains 19 amino acids including the essentials. In many countries, vegetarians are advised to supplement their intake of vegetables and fruits with Chlorella pyrenoidosa. The commonly used consumption of meat and milk products is one of the major contributory risks and causes of cancer, heart disease, osteoporosis, obesity and diabetes. The individual amino acids have many good qualities. They can be used to both prevent and treat disease states in a biological way without the risk of serious side effects.

Leucine
Leucine helps in regulating blood sugar levels, growth and repair of muscle tissues, (body bones, skin and muscles), growth hormone production, wound healing, and energy change.
Leucine is used in the biosynthesis of proteins.
Leucine may help prevent muscle protein degradation, which sometimes occurs after trauma or severe stress.
Leucine may also be beneficial to individuals suffering from a condition that he or she can not metabolize the amino acid phenylalanine.

Deficiency of leucine is rare as all food with proteins contains this amino acid, but vegans and vegetarians without sufficient protein sources, can suffer shortcomings of this amino acid that can cause symptoms like dizziness, fatigue, headache, irritation and other problems.

Valine

Valine has a stimulating effect and is important for muscle metabolism, repair and growth of tissues and maintenance of the nitrogen balance in the body. Because it is a chain-branched amino acid, it can be used as an energy source in muscles and thus protects the glucose function. A lack of amino acids can occur when using drugs, and valine plays an important role and there is a suggestion that it may also be beneficial in the treatment of alcohol-related brain damage as well as degenerative neurological conditions.

Lysine

Lysine is required for growth and bone development in children, assisting in calcium absorption and is important for maintaining proper nitrogen balance in the body. Furthermore, lysine is important for the production of antibodies, hormones, enzymes, collagen formation as well as repair of tissues.

Since lysine helps build muscle protein, it is important for patients to recover after injury, recover after surgery and also for the maintenance of healthy blood vessels.

Lysine also appears to support the fight against herpes and inflammations. Although rarely present, because there are many protein sources, lack of lysine may cause symptoms such as anaemia, enzyme disorder, lack of energy , hair loss, weight loss and delayed growth, as well as reproductive problems, poor appetite and impaired concentration.

Threonine

Threonine helps to maintain the correct protein balance in the body as well as assisting the formation of collagen and elastin.

In addition, threonine is important for liver function also to counteract fatty liver, in combination with aspartic acid and methionine as well as assisting the immune system by supporting the production of antibodies and promoting thyme growth and activity. Other nutrients are more easily absorbed in the presence of threonine, which has also been used as part of mental health treatment. A lack of threonine can result in irritability and a generally impaired personality change.

Phenylalanine
Phenylalanine is appetite suppressant and therefore useful for persons who want to lose weight. It is also stimulating for your mood because it is so closely linked to the nervous system and, in addition, phenylalanine is a promotion for memory and learning. People suffering from Parkinson's disease are recommended to take phenylalanine.

Methionine
Methionine assists in fat degradation, thus preventing formation of fat in the arteries as well as promoting the digestive system.
Methionine helps to remove heavy metals from the body because it is converted to cysteine which is precursor to glutathione which in turn is important for detoxification of the liver.
Amino acid methionine is also an important antioxidant as the sulfur it delivers disables free radicals.
Methionine is also used in the treatment of depression, pain by arthritis as well as in chronic liver disease, even though these claims are still under investigation.

Methionine is a part of the three amino acids necessary for the body to produce creatine mono-hydrate, a
composition that is of major importance for energy
production and muscle building.
Large deficiency of methionine can be manifested in
dementia, while at lower deficiency you may experience symptoms such as fatty liver, slow growth, weak-
ness, edema and skin problems.

Isoleucine
Isoleucine participates in promoting muscle strength
recovery after physical exertion, and important for the
formation of hemoglobin as well as being helpful in
regulating blood glucose levels and energy levels.
Lack of isoleucine is most common in people who
suffer from protein deficiency with symptoms which
lead to headache, dizziness, fatigue, depression,
confusion and irritation.

Tryptophan
Tryptophan is required for the production of niacin
(vitamin B3).
This amino acid is used by the body to produce serotonin, a neurotransmitter which is important for normal nerve and brain functions. Serotonin is important
for sleep, pain control, more stable mood, inflammation, bowel movements etc.
Tryptophan is also important for controlling hyperactivity in children, stress relief, weight loss and appetite reduction.
It has also been shown that people suffering from
migraines are in short supply and therefore are having
a good reason to receive supplementation of tryptophan.

Lack of this amino acid in combination with magnesium deficiency can be a contributory cause of cardiac arteries spasms.

Chlorella's other amino acids

Histidine
Histidine is also a precursor of histamine, a tissue hormone secreted from mast cells in certain allergic
reactions. Histidine is important for the growth and
repair of tissues as well as the preservation of myelin
skids (lipid-rich isolation around the nerves that
protect them and which breaks down when multiple
sclerosis occurs). Histidine is also important for the
production of red and white blood cells and helps
protect the body from radiation damage and contributes to the removal of heavy metals.

Histidine promotes the production of gastric juices
and people with a shortage of these and who suffer
from poor combustion, may also benefit from this
nutrient.

In addition, it has been reported that an increased intake of histidine may contribute to prolonged orgasm
and also provide more intense sexual pleasure.

Arginine
Arginine is very important when it comes to the improvement of the immune system and increases the
size and activity of the thymus gland responsible for
the production of T-lymphocytes - the so called T-cells
that promote the immune system. For this reason,
Arginine may be suitable for people suffering from
AIDS or other malignant diseases which suppress the
immune system.

In the pancreas, arginine is used to release insulin and in the pituitary gland, this amino acid is a component of human growth hormone, which also contributes to sexual stimulation (prolonged orgasm). Arginine is important for the health of the liver through the help of being able to neutralize ammonia in the liver. It is also involved in the condition of the skin and tissues - healing and repair of tissues as well as the formation of collagen.

Arginine occurs in sperm and L-Arginine is used in the treatment of the male's sexual health and has also been used in the treatment of sterility. Arginine is important for muscle metabolism, retention of nitrogen balance as well as weight control, as it facilitates increase of muscle mass while decreasing body fat. As a deficiency indication (though rare), impairment of insulin production and hair loss may be mentioned.

Aspartic acid

Aspartic acid is of the utmost importance for metabolism produced by other amino acids and biochemicals. Among the latter being synthesized from aspartic acid, are asparagine, arginine, lysine, methionine, threonine, isoleucine and several nucleotides (molecules composed by a purine or pyrimidine, a group of sugars and at least one phosphate group.

Nucleotides are building blocks by which nucleic acids as DNA and RNA are build up.

A lack of aspartic acid can show symptoms like fatigue and depression.

Glutamic acid

Glutamic acid is an important neurotransmitter and also important for the metabolism of sugars and fats. Glutamic acid helps in the transport of potassium across the blood brain barrier (the barrier between the brain and the bloodstream) although it itself does not pass this barrier so easily. Glutamic acid shows good signs that make an important contribution in future treatment of neurological conditions, wounds, muscular dystrophy, epilepsy, Parkinson's disease and mental retardation (reduced intelligence).

Glutamic acid can be used as fuel for the brain and can be attached to the nitrogen atoms in the process of production of glutamine and this activity also detoxifies the body from ammonia.

This activity is the only way in which the brain is detoxified from ammonia.

The liquid produced by the prostate gland also contains a variety of glutamic acid and can therefore play an important role.

Proline

Proline is one of the cyclic amino acids that are a major component of the protein collagen, the connective tissue structure that connects and supports all other tissues.

Glycine

Glycine is needed for the development of protein in the body and nucleic synthesis, production of RNA and DNA, bile acids and other amino acids in the body. It has also proved to be contributing to the absorption of calcium in the body. Glycine supports the inhibition of muscle degeneration as it helps to deliver extra creatine to the body.

Glycine occurs in quite large amounts in the prostate fluid and, for that reason, it may be important for prostate health. Amino acid glycine, which is also used by the nervous system and its function as an inhibitory neurotransmitter, plays a role in the prevention of epileptic seizures and is also used in the treatment of manic depression and hyperactivity.

Deficiency: Few people show a lack of glycine, partly because the body itself makes the non-essential amino acid and partly because the diet contains large amounts of it.

Cystine

Cysteine is required for the skin as well as for the detoxification of the body. Cysteine is present in beta-carotene, the major protein in nails, skin and hair.
It is not only important in collagen production but also promotes skin elasticity and texture. The need for cysteine is important to the production of the amino acid taurine and is a component of the antioxidant glutathione.

Cysteine is useful in detoxifying the body of harmful substances and to guard the brain and liver from alcohol damage. It has also been found that cysteine has a tonic effect on the stomach and intestines that can be helpful to prevent damage caused by the ingestion of aspirin and similar drugs.

Cysteine is also essential for the metabolism of a number of necessary biochemicals include coenzyme A, heparin, biotin and glutathione.

Ornithine
Ornithine is important because it releases growth hormone in the body which, in turn, helps with fat metabolism. It is also important for a normal functioning of the immune system and helps to detoxify and restore the liver from ammonia.

Ornithine has a repairing and healing effect on skin and tissues in which body parts one find this amino acid.
Lack of Ornithine occurs rarely because the body itself produces this amino acid which is not essential.

CHLORELLA VITAMINS

Vitamin A and beta carotene.

As previously mentioned, chlorella contains a variety of nutrition in all natural and organic forms.
One of the most important of these is pro-vitamin A, the form of vitamin A that is most easily digested and which can not be built up to toxic levels in the body.
After protein deficiency, vitamin-A deficiency is most common on Earth.
   Vitamin A regulates the immune system that helps prevent infection by producing white blood cells that destroy harmful bacteria and virus.
Vitamin A can also help lymphocytes (a type of white blood cells) to fight infection more effectively.

Generally, there are two categories of vitamin A, depending on whether the source of nutrition is from animal or plant kingdom.
Vitamin-A is in the form of retinol (from animal kingdom) and in the form of beta carotene (from the plant kingdom).
There is no need for a daily vitamin A intake because this vitamin is stored in the liver and adipose tissues to be used later by the body when needed. Today it is important to use a appropriate source of vitamin A as this substance is reduced in the body through a num-ber of environmental factors.

For example, vitamin A can be prevented from being assimilated and stored in the body already at low exposure levels of pesticides.

Dr Saffioti, a director at the National Cancer, Institute, reported at the ninth International Cancer Congress, that vitamin A can help prevent lung cancer. Vitamin A is also important for the development of a fetus, so make sure there is enough vitamin A in the breast milk when breastfeeding.

As an addition, it can be mentioned that vitamin A is important for the child's growth. Vitamin A is important for the cells of the skin and the mucous membranes of the bowel, eyes, respiratory organs and urinary tract mucous membranes as well as being an important protection against infection and the development of some cancers.

Vitamin A regulates the immune system and helps prevent infection by producing white blood cells that destroy harmful bacteria and various viruses.

Vitamin A deficiency:
*Decreased night vision, night blindness.
*Dry mucous membranes that can be easily infected
*Increased risk of skin cancer, bronchus and stomach.
*Impaired quality of hair and nails
*Dry skin that flakes easily.

It rarely occurs an overdose. It occurs acute overdose at doses of 100-500 mg.
Pregnant women should not exceed a daily dose of 3 mg. Symptoms of overdose could be severe headache, flaky and dry skin, joint pain, nausea, vomiting and constipation.

One should keep in mind that vitamin interacts with zinc why a lack of the latter may reduce the effect of vitamin A and vice versa.
Women who use birth control pills have less need for vitamin A and young people who use vitamin A cream for acne should not eat extra of vitamin A.

Vitamin A occurs in liver, egg, butter, margarine, cheese, mackerel and sardines.

In Chlorella vitamin A occurs in the form of provitamin A (carotenoid) that is converted to vitamin A into the intestines using bile salts, thyroid hormone and shortening.

Vitamin A is formed in the liver and intestinal walls of provitamin A (carotenoids). Beta carotene is a plant substance that the body converts to vitamin A. One tablespoon Chlorella provides the body with about 200% of the daily minimum vitamin-A requirement namely in its safest and completely natural form such as pro-vitamin A.
100 grams of Chlorella contain 180 mg beta-carotene. Beta-carotene has the greatest vitamin A activity and antioxidant activity of all carotenoids.

When degradative processes in the body release free radicals in the form of unstable oxygen atoms, beta carotene prevents these atoms from joining other substances into harmful oxides. Beta carotene also prevents other free radicals from initiating harmful processes in organisms.
Beta carotene, such as that of Chlorella, in all natural forms, also protects against the oxidation process caused by light. People with sensitive skin can get extra protection by using beta carotene.

Beta carotene in natural form has been shown to prevent the development of cancerous cells and, in addition, to intensify macrophage production of tumor necrosis factor (TNF) and T-cell stimulator interleukin I.
It has been found that people who eat low beta carotene diets are more at risk of developing lung cancer, stomach cancer, prostate cancer and cervical cancer. As an antioxidant, beta carotene acts as a complement to antioxidant substances such as vitamins C and E, as well as the catalytic and glutathione peroxidase enzymes. Beta carotene works synergistically with vitamin E as an antioxidant to kill cancer cells at its early stage.

Chlorella contains more beta carotene and lutein than most green and yellow vegetables. This micro algae is a particularly rich source of lutein, a powerful full antioxidant, known to be particularly beneficial to the eyes. These natural pigments are absorbed through the digestive system and can therefore be expected to be fully effective. Lutein is known to protect against problems such as cataracts, macular degeneration (age changes in the yellow spot) and retinal problems.
        Researchers at the Department of Nutritional Sciences at the University of Wisconsin, USA, show the importance of lutein to prevent the extent of age-related cataracts in adults, 50-86 years old, being the only carotenoid of 5 tested which proved to be protective against the development of cataract. (Lyle)
Some species of chlorella contain 50 times more lutein than spinach.

The doctors Joel Schwartz, Diana Suda and Gerald Shklar of Harvard School of Dental Medicine presented this research result at the 1986 Academy at Oral Pathology, Toronto, Canada. They also pointed out that studies of Chlorella extracts proved more effective than only the beta carotene, which allowed the group of researchers to speculate that other substances may be present in the algae which give greater anti-tumor effect than the actual beta carotene content. (Hixson. J.R: Beta-Carotene showing promise as topical agent. Medical Tribune August 6, 1986, p.3)

VITAMIN B

B-vitamins are a group of water-soluble vitamins that have the same effects and importance. These vitamins are taken up and excreted rapidly in the body and therefore we need to eat the B-vitamins every day. One exception is vitamin B12, which is stored in our liver.
In chlorella, we find the B-vitamins together in a complex and not broken down into individual B-vitamins.
   They cooperate with each other in a chain of chemical enzyme reactions in which each B-vitamin works as part-enzyme.
More of B-vitamins have a preserving effect on the organism and therefore function as antioxidants. E-vitamins protect the body against environmental pollutants and the more polluted environment we live in, the more B-vitamins we need in the diet.

Vitamin-B1 (thiamine)

Thiamine was the first time, discovered in 1910 by Umetaro Suzuki in Japan, when he examined the relationship of substances in rice bran that cured patients suffering from Beri Beri.

In 1926, vitamin B1 was isolated from rice bran and in 1936 an American synthesized vitamin B1, after which it was named thiamine. Thiamine also known as vitamin B1, is a water soluble vitamin commonly found in most foods.

Like most of the B-vitamins, thiamine plays a role in how our body uses energy from food and is vital for cellular function.

Thiamine specifically helps the body convert carbohydrates to energy that is important for metabolism, focus and strength.

Vitamin B1 contributes to good digestion and is sometimes called nerve vitamin as it has a positive effect on the nervous system and the brain (memory, depression, sleeping difficulty).

Vitamin B1 is considered to be an important antioxidant that can prevent damage by oxidation in the cells. The risk of deficiency symptoms increases when we are consuming a lot of sweets and drink too much coffee, tea and alcohol.

Vitamin B1 is recommended to young people living on sugar and empty calories, pregnant and nursing mothers and the elderly and diabetic patients.

Thiamine B1 deficiency is caused by consuming a diet low in animal products and overconsumption of alcohol.

The most common vitamin B1 deficiency symptoms include:

Chronic fatigue, gut issues, muscle wasting, neurological neurological degeneration.

It also plays a role in healthy liver function and is needed for healthy skin, eyes, hair, and nails. Most foods are a good source of thiamine.

The RDA for thiamine is 1.2 mg/day for men and 1.1 mg/day for women. Chlorella contains around 15 mg vitamin B1 per 100 g.

Vitamin B2 (riboflavin)
Vitamin-B2 is readily absorbed, water-soluble micro-nutrient that also promote energy metabolism. Riboflavin was discovered in 1920, isolated in 1933, and first made in 1935. It is on the World Health Organization List of Essential Medicines as the most important medications needed in a basic health system. Riboflavin is in the vitamin B-group. Vitamin B2 is necessary for the body for cellular respiration.
Food sources include eggs, green vegetables, milk, and meat.
The vitamin is essential for the formation of red blood cells and breathing mixture, antibody production and regulation of the human growth and reproduction. It is important for skin, nails, hair growth and good health in general, which also includes the regulation of thyroid activity.
Riboflavin also helps to prevent or treat various types of eye problems, including cataract.
Exposure to light destroys riboflavin in cheese, milk, leafy vegetables, liver and yeast, which otherwise is a good source of this vitamin.
Riboflavin deficiency results in stomatitis including painful red tongue, sore throat, chapped and fissured lips and inflammation of the corners of the mouth.
It can be oily scaly skin rashes on the scrotum, vulva and sores of the lip.

The eyes can become itchy, watery, bloodshot and sensitive to light. Due to interference with iron absorption, even mild to moderate riboflavin deficiency results in an anaemia with normal cell size and normal haemoglobin content (i.e., normochromic anaemia). This is distinct from anaemia caused by deficiency of folic acid (B9) or cyanocobalamin (B12), which causes anaemia with large blood cells (megaloblastic anaemia).

Deficiency of riboflavin during pregnancy can result in birth defects including congenital heart defects and limb deformities
Lack of riboflavin is manifested in cold sores, dry and sore lips, inflammation of the mucous membranes (cracks in the corners of the mouth), the tongue and the skin (nose and scrotum). In light deficiency can feel tired and weak, get brittle nails and hair loss and dry, itchy eyes.

Chlorella generally contains 4.8 mg of vitamin B2 per 100 grams.

Vitamin B3 (niacin and niacin amide)
Niacin is required for the metabolism of carbohydrates and fats as well as proteins. Niacin appears as acid (nicotinic acid) and as amide (nicotinamide), is water soluble and must therefore be administered to the body daily.
Serious deficiency of the vitamin can cause pellagra deficiency. B is important in the formation of sex hormones such as estrogen, progesterone and testosterone, and also increases the pain threshold.
A daily intake of more than 22 mg of niacin can pro-tect against the development of Alzheimer's disease and the cognitive degradation associated with older people.

Vitamin B3 occurs in fish, beer yeast, peanuts, graham flour, fruit, nuts, vegetables, potatoes and eggs. Chlorella contains about 28 mg of vitamin B3 per 100 g.

Vitamin B5 (Pantothenic acid)

Pantothenic acid is water soluble and is needed for good health in general. Pantothenic acid is necessary for the combustion of amino acids and carbohydrates, and in particular in connection with fat metabolism and cholesterol, as well as for the hormones and other important substances associated with cholesterol.

Pantothenic acid is also recommended for elderly people who have poor eating habits as well as for pregnant and breastfeeding. To note is that panto-thenic acid can improve the effect of medicines for chronic diseases, eg. Parkinson's disease and senility (Alzheimer's).

Vitamin B5 (pantothenic acid) occurs in brewers yeast, bananas, wheat germs, pork liver, fish, nuts, meat, avocado, fruit, berries, and egg and milk products. Chlorella contains about 15 mg of pantothenic acid per 100 g.

Vitamin B6 (pyridoxine)

Pyridoxine is formed from three active substances (pyridoxin, pyridoxal and pyridoxamine). Pyridoxine assists the balance between sodium and potassium and also promotes the production of red blood cells.

Vitamin B6 is associated with cancer immunity and helps combat homocysteine formation.

Pyridoxine is water-soluble and is not sensitive to low heat but is sensitive to light. Deep-freezing of vegetables reduces vitamin B6 content as well as heat preservation.

Pyridoxine is involved in synthesizing the DNA/RNA and is a cofactor of the enzyme that helps to convert tryptophan to serotonin and L-dopa to dopamine. This vitamin plays an important role in normal pregnancy.
It has also been mentioned in connection with children who have difficulty learning and can also help prevent eczema and psoriasis.
Pyridoxine can help balance hormone changes in woman and stimulate the immune system. Lack of pyridoxine can cause anaemia, nerve damage, skin problems and sore on the lips.
Chlorella generally contains about 16 mg vitamin B6 per 100 g.

Biotin (B7)
Biotin is a water soluble vitamin and is produced in the body by different special intestinal bacteria and may also be fed through the food. Biotin is necessary for metabolism of carbohydrates, fat and amino acids, (protein building blocks). Biotin is necessary for both metabolism and growth in humans with regard to the production of fatty acids, antibodies, digestive enzymes and metabolism of niacin (Vitamin B3). It is relatively uncommon with a lack of biotin, but in that case, it can lead to hair loss, dry skin, dry eyes, cracks in the corners of the mouths, loss of appetite, fatigue, insomnia and depression. Biotin is found in liver, kidney, soya and egg yolks.
Chlorella generally contains 313 µg biotin (B7) per 100 grams

Vitamin B12 (cobalamin)
Vitamin B_{12}, also called cobalamin, is a water-soluble vitamin that has a key role in the normal functioning of the brain and nervous system via the synthesis

of myelin (myelinogenesis), and the formation of red blood cells. It is one of eight B vitamins. It is involved in the metabolism of every cell of the human body, especially affecting DNA synthesis, fatty acid and amino acid metabolism. No fungi, plants, or animals (including humans) are capable of producing vitamin B12.

Recommended daily intake of vitamin B12 is 5-7 ug. Vitamin B12 is naturally found in meat (especially in liver), shellfish, eggs and dairy products.

Chlorella, which has an easily absorbable content of vitamin B12 is recommended for vegetarians. This vitamin differs from other B-vitamins as it forms in the intestine through microorganism and is stored in the liver. A substance in the stomach's intrinsic mucosa is required for the vitamin B12 to be taken up from the intestine. A sick mucous membrane can lead to vitamin B12 deficiency.

Deficiency of B12 may cause greater risk of losing bone mass in older women, and according to recent research, also increasing the risk of dementia Alzheimer's disease.

Anaemia occurs when your blood doesn't carry enough oxygen to the rest of your body.

PABA (para-aminobenzoic acid) (B10)

PABA (B10) is manufactured by the intestines of humans. PABA helps the good bacteria to make folic acid, supports the formation of red blood cells and contains sunscreening properties.

Lack of PABA can lead to extreme fatigue, eczema, irritation, pressure, nervousness, constipation, headache and digestive problems.

Choline

Choline is very important in the control of fat and building of cholesterol in the body, preventing fat from accumulation in the liver, facilitates the fat balance in the cells, regulates the kidneys, liver, and gall bladder and is important for the nervous system and stimulates memory. Lack of choline can lead to fatty liver and liver cirrhosis over time, arteriosclerosis, heart problems, high blood pressure and renal haemorrhage.

Folic acid (vitamin B9)

Folic acid is water soluble and belongs to the vitamin B family. Folic acid is important for protein metabolism and especially during pregnancy, it is important to take folic acid. Folic acid is necessary for the production of genetic material DNA/RNA and red blood cells, healing wounds as well as production of muscle tissue.
Folic acid works intimately with vitamins B6 and B12 and protects against cardiac problems by controlling blood levels in homocysteine, which is a byproduct of protein metabolism.
Vitamin B has established effects to reduce depression levels. Chlorella generally contains 15 mg folic acid per 100 grams.

Inositol (Vitamin Bh)

Inositol is a water-soluble member of the Vitamin B family. This vitamin is necessary for proper compilation of cell membranes.
Inositol affects the nerve transmission, and supports the transport of fat in the body.
Inositol is used primarily in the treatment of liver problems, depression and diabetes.
Inositol also helps with degradation of fat. Inositol is not really a vitamin but interacts with many vitamins

and other nutrients. Low levels of inositol may cause depression, and in many cases attention has been drawn to the fact that inositol intake can instead counteract the depressions. Serotonin requires inositol for better functioning.
Chlorella generally contains 198.5 mg inositol per 100 g.

Vitamin C (ascorbic acid)
This vitamin is water soluble and is considered important for our lives and maintaining good health. The strength of the vitamin is lost when exposed to air, light and heat. Most animals synthesize their own vitamin C.

There are some exceptions such as man and monkey. The main function of vitamin C is to strengthen the immune system and thus to increase the resistance to infections, flu, colds and cancer. Vitamin C is important in the formation of connective tissue collagen. This applies primarily to bone tissue, teeth and cartilage. Vitamin C is necessary for the production of a variety of hormones and the body's own analgesic, endorphin.

Vitamin C is an important antioxidant. Deficiencies can occur such as allergy, fatigue, reduced defenses against infections and impaired sore healing, muscle weaknesses, skin bleeding, bruising and elevated blood cholesterol, loss of appetite, anaemia and digestive problems. C-Vitamin deficiency can also be expected to increase the risk of cancer and cardio-vascular disease.

Chlorella contains about 50 mg vitamin C per 100 g.

Vitamin D (calciferol)

Vitamin D is a fat-soluble vitamin (hormone) and proves to be stable to heat. It is actually a hormone and very important for the good health of your body. Vitamin D is present in small portions in food, but can be formed primarily by the sun's ultraviolet rays. That is why it is so important to eat chlorella being cultured in outside pools!

The liver and kidneys help to convert vitamin D into its active hormonal form. The main biological function in vitamin D facilitates absorption and the use of calcium and phosphorus. Vitamin D is important for the formation of teeth and bones, making good balance of the nervous system and the heart's activity. Most importantly, vitamin D is important for osteoporosis, which is a major problem, not least in populations such as in low-fat countries and will mostly occur in women, also by hormonal unbalances.

Contemporary research has shown the importance of vitamin D in the fight against cancer, diabetes, arthritis, infertility and PMS.

Vitamin D deficiency has also been mentioned in connection with obesity as it has been shown that the vitamin reduces leptin secretion. Leptin is a hormone produced by fat cells and is involved with our weight regulation. It is thought that the hormone signals to the brain as the fat cells are "full".

Vitamin D is directly associated with Syndrome X, which has occurred in a problem group that includes insulin resistance (inability to take care of carbohydrates in the diet), abnormal blood fats such as elevated cholesterol levels and triglyceride levels, overweight and high blood pressure.

Chlorella pyrenoidosa contains about 37000IE of vitamin D in natural form per 100 grams.

Vitamin E (a-tocopherol)

Vitamin E consists of a family of eight fat-soluble substances.the most active form which also is the most common in our diet of all, is called alphatoco-pherol.

Vitamin E is one of the most important vitamins being able to defending us against free radicals. Free radicals can cause cellular damage that can contribute to the development of heart disease and cancer. E vitamin also helps to protect other antioxidants and can pro-tect us against various diseases as stroke, arthritis, senility, diabetes and cancer.

Vitamin E delays cellular aging due to oxidation by adding oxygen to the blood, which then passes to the heart and other organs, nourishes cells, strengthens the capillary walls, and protects the red blood cells from degrading toxins as well as prevents and eliminates blood clots.

Vitamin E contributes regulation of our central nervous system and the balance between progesterone and estrogen.

Vitamin E increases the concentration of the good cholesterol HDL which prevents atherosclerosis.

The healing power of tocopherols is often linked to that of vitamin C and another antioxidant (sister oxidant) that actually increases the effectiveness of vitamin E.

The combination promises good help in preventing complications such as some heart problems, alcohol problems, cancer, HIV infection and MS.

Chlorella has generally 11 mg per 100g of vitamin E

Phylloquinone (Vitamin K1),
Vitamin K or phylloquinone, is a vitamin found in food and used as a dietary supplement. As a supplement it is used to treat certain bleeding disorders like overdose of Warfarin, vitamin K deficiency and by obstructive jaundice. Vitamin K is also recommended to prevent and treat hemorrhagic disease of the newborn.

Vitamin K is fat-soluble and is important for protein synthesis and necessary for blood coagulation. Normally the vitamin is produced by bowel bacteria and lack of this vitamin occurs very rarely except in cases of damaged intestines.
Vitamin K prevents calcification in the arteries and other soft tissues.
Chlorella generally contains 711 ug of K1 vitamin per 100 g.

Chlorella Minerals
Mineral substances are vital for our body and are essential nutrients needed to regulate many bodily functions. Two types of minerals are used, partly those called macro minerals or only minerals and partly those called trace substances.
Macro-minerals are calcium, magnesium phosphorus, sodium, sulphur, chlorine and potassium.
        The trace elements include zinc, iron, copper, chromium, manganese, iodine and selenium. The minerals have many important tasks for our body.

Calcium
Calcium account for around 1% - 2% of adult human body weight and over 99% is found in teeth and bones.

Calcium is best known for its role in developing and maintaining our skeleton and teeth.
It strengthens the heart, bones and teeth and prevents acidification of the body. Calcium, phosphorus, magnesium and vitamin D work together to counteract osteoporosis. Many women take extra doses of calcium and vitamin D in hopes of preventing osteoporosis. Calcium deficiency causes fragile and soft skeleton, tooth decay, rickets, impaired bone formation and bleeding.

Calcium is recommended:
* during pregnancy and lactation,
* low calcium diet
* bone breakage,
* diarrheas with decreased absorption
* diabetes
* alcoholism
* kidney disease with increased secretion
* nervousness and sleep insomnia
* high blood pressure
* problems with hair and nails (fragile)
* osteoporosis
* bleeding gums
Chlorella generally contains 350 mg per 100 grams of calcium.

Potassium (K)
Potassium is important for the function of the cells, as well as for kidneys, muscles and maintenance of good heartbeat stroke and regulation of acid/base balance. The nervous cells contain a lot of potassium. Signs of potassium deficiency may be irregular pulse and weak muscle strength in both leg muscles (paralysis) and the intestine which may cause constipation.

Another sign of potassium deficiency may be numbness in arms and legs.
Chlorella is rich in potassium with a general content of about 1,300 milligrams per 100 grams.

Phosphor (P)

Phosphorus is the most common mineral in addition to calcium in the body. Phosphorus is important for bone and teeth, energy metabolism and for the body's acid-base balance. Phosphorus occurs in excessive quantities in household foods such as meat, chicken, fish, egg, nuts, whole grain and soft drinks. Too much phosphorus can bind salt and make the body sour. Fruits and vegetables as well as Chlorella have good phosphorus/calcium balance

Magnesium (Mg)

Magnesium regulates acid/base balance, promotes cell renewal, weight retention, muscles and is important to the nervous system. Magnesium prevents constipation, activates enzymes and participates in many chemical processes and is therefore very important. Magnesium deficiency occurs to a large extent by the population, not least because of a one-sided, low-magnesium diet. Lack of magnesium may cause irregular heartbeat, signs of angina and osteoporosis.

In chlorella you find magnesium generally of about 316 mg per 100 grams.

Manganese (Mn)

Human consumption of manganese occurs mainly through food such as spinach, tea and herbs, soya beans, nuts, olive oil, green beans and oysters.

After absorption in the body, the manganese is transported through the blood to the liver, kidney, pancreas and to the endocrine glands.
Manganese helps to form hemoglobin, activate enzymes and improve the memory. In the absence of manganese, the following symptoms may occur:

* overweight
* glucose intolerance
* blood clots
* skin problems
* skeletal disorders
* birth defects
* hair color changes
* nerve problems

Chlorella content of manganese is 5,5 mg per 100 gram.

Cobalt (Co)
The highest levels of traces of cobalt are found in the heart, kidneys, liver and bone tissue and excretion occurs though the urine.
Cobalt is recommended for vegetarians who do not eat fish that contains a lot of cobalt.
Cobalt affects blood pressure and the thyroid gland. In the absence of cobalt, goître may occur.
There are traces of cobalt in chlorella.

Iron (Fe)
Iron is important for functions of the red blood cells which also includes the formation and acidification of the tissues. Most iron is found in the red blood cells. It helps to form hemoglobin and insufficient intake of iron in the diet may cause anemia.

On the other hand, the cause of anemia may be lack of magnesium, zinc or copper. Iron improves blood quality and helps the body to prevent infections by strengthening the body's resistance.
Risk of iron deficiency can occur in the case of over-consumption of milk products, bread and sausages, vegan diet and often happens for lactose vegetarians.
Iron deficiency can also occur during menstrual bleeding, pregnancy, breastfeeding and lactation, stomach ulcer, hemorrhoids, cancer, long-term infections and candida. Intake of vitamin C helps the body to absorb iron more easily.
Chlorella contains about 205 mg iron per 100 grams.

Copper (Cu)
Copper is an important trace element for both human and animals.
Lack of copper can lead to anaemia, osteoporosis, neurophilic (abnormally low levels of white blood cells). Copper is important for enzymes that form cholesterol.
Another important task of copper is to contribute to a strong cardiovascular system.
Prolonged lack of copper can lead to elevated levels of cholesterol, weak blood vessels and enlarged heart.
The richest sources of copper are nuts, legumes, liver, kidney, seafood, and oysters.
Lack of copper can lead to heart problems, hypertension and weakened immune system.

In Chlorella copper is generally found to be about 0.06 mg per 100 g

Selenium (Sc)
Selenium is an important trace element and anti-oxidant which are considered to be vital for health in total. Selenium increases HDL, the good cholesterol and strengthens the cells in the fight against cancer (anti mutagenic). Selenium can be found among others in eggs, meat and fish. Liver is especially rich in selenium. Recommended daily intake is 55 micro-grams. More studies have shown that there is a correlation between cancer and lack of selenium.
There has also been discovered lower levels of selenium in patients with AIDS. Deficiency of selenium causes deflation of the immune system.
Chlorella contains approximately 0.8ug organic selenium per 100 grams.

Sulphur
The largest concentration of sulphur is found in the skin and in the cartilage, and excreted in the urine.
Sulphur relieves dermatitis and eczema, promotes the compilation of proteins and the ionic balance of the tissues.
Lack of sulphur is quite unknown as we get sulphur in meat, eggs, vegetables and dairy products, soybeans, tofu and green vegetables, peas, cabbage, onions, potatoes, carrots, celery, asparagus, avocados, and radishes.
Chlorella contains traces of sulphur.

Zinc (Zn)
Zinc is a vital substance and an important anti-oxidant and for the production of new cells as well as for the enzyme function.
For men it is particularly important with zinc in con-nection with prostate enlargement.

Prostate is the organ that has the greatest need for this mineral and it is also of great interest to the immune system. It is important to take zinc together with vitamin B6 as lack of the latter can cause extra zinc secretion from the body.

Reduction of zinc in the blood is often associated with, among other things, infections, malignant tumors, leukemia, liver disease and anaemia and reduced metabolism. P-pills can be a common cause of zinc deficiency in women. Zinc occurs among other things in nuts, wheat germs, beans, sunflower seeds, wheat bran, meat, spices, eggs, pineapples, potatoes and carrots.

Chlorella generally contains 66 mg per 100 g of natural mineral zinc.

Sodium (Na)

The most important task for sodium is that this mineral along with chlorine can preserve the osmotic pressure in the body fluids. Lack of sodium may occur in connection with diarrhea, vomiting, and also in severe sweating. Sodium maintains the balance between calcium and potassium, regulates body fluids and stimulates digestion.

Some good sources of sodium are asparagus, cucumber, celery, carrots, figs, cabbage and oatmeal.

Chlorella contains generally 29 mg sodium per 100 g.

Iodine

Iodine is considered to be a vital trace element. Its most important function in humans is to participate in the production of thyroxine which is the thyroid hormone.

This hormone participates in controlling the metabolic process in all the body's cells and organs. Lack of iodine can cause goitre. The main sources of iodine are dairy products and fish. There are also small amounts of iodine in eggs, meat and bread.
In general, chlorella contains about 0.6 mg iodine per 100 grams.

Essential fatty acids
we need fatty substances to maintain good health. There are about 20 fatty acids that are important to the body's normal functions. Two of these can't be synthesized by our bodies and are therefore called essential fatty acids.
Alpha-linolenic acid (ALA), omega-3 fatty acid and omega-6 fatty acid should be in right balance in our diet. Essential fatty acids act as building blocks for all cell membranes in the body.
They produce prostaglandins that are tissue hormones, necessary for energy metabolism, the heart and for the immune system. The essential fatty acids compete with the poor fats (trans-fats), why it is important to minimize the intake of trans-fats, LDL-cholesterol and instead eat more of the good and useful fats.

The essential fats (beneficial fats) raise HDL, the good cholesterol, which, in turn, escorts the the poor cholesterol LDL to the liver where it is broken down and removed.
This is even more important now when so many people struggle to lower their bad cholesterol and prevent cardiovascular disease and fatness.
Essential fatty acids (EFAs) assist the cardiovascular system, reproductive system, immune system, and nervous system.

The human body needs these fatty acids to make and repair cell membranes that allow the cells to get optimal nutrition so that they can dispose of hazardous waste products.

Deficiency increases the risk of atherosclerosis and cardiovascular disease, increased premenstrual syndrome (PMS) and disease of the nervous system, including multiple sclerosis.

Chlorella generally contains 3200 mg linolenic acid (omega-3) and 2800 mg linoleic acid (omega-6) per 100 grams.
Chlorella also contains 11 other fatty acids.

Average composition of fat in chlorella:
Total unsaturated fats: 81.8%   *   Total saturated fat 18.2%

Carbohydrates
Carbohydrates are vital to humans. It provides fuel to the body, good fuel if you choose the right food.
Carbohydrates are found in the diet, among other things in bread, beans, milk, potatoes, spaghetti, and wheat.
Green plants, for example chlorella, uses photosynthesis to combine carbon dioxide and water to form carbohydrates.
Carbohydrates can be stored in the liver and muscles using inulin and cortisol (steroid hormone).

Glucose is found in all fruits and vegetables. Glucose is readily absorbed in the blood and delivered to the cells in all organs, glands, tissues and body systems and trans-formed into energy. The brain uses about 25% of glucose, or blood sugar.

Complex carbohydrates are broken down into single sugar by the enzymes activity. Most fruits and vegetables are classified as complex carbohydrates such as, for example, potatoes.
The main benefit of these carbohydrates is that they still provide current of sugar blood, which stabilizes energy production and show gentle caution with the pancreas.
Chlorella contains about 20% carbohydrates.

Albumin
Japanese researchers have recently found that chlorella can raise blood levels of the protein albumin.
Albumin is one of the most powerful antioxidants in the body, as well as its most important transport system that delivers vitamins, minerals, fatty acids, hormones and other essential substances throughout the body.
Albumin is also a tool for removing toxins from cells into the liver where they break down and are later extracted from the body.
   Without adequate levels of albumin, neither kidneys, liver and other vital organs can do their work and the immune system can't work efficiently.
A variety of studies have shown that a low albumin level is a marker of serious disease such as cancer and heart disease.
This discovery is underlined by a breakthrough for a British cardiac study, published in The Lancet, in which 7735 middle aged men were checked for more than 9 years.
The researchers found that men with the lowest level of albumin showed the highest death rate caused by several different diseases, including heart disease.

Our album level drops with age, which is an indication that albumin can play an important role in trying to keep our body healthy, strong and youthful.
Smokers generally have lower album levels. It is not surprising that researchers believe that increase of albumin can have a healthy effect.
They point to the studies performed, confirming that a level increase of albumin can both prevent cancer changes and prolong the life span of human cells.

CGF (Chlorella Growth Factor)
The most interesting content of chlorella is an ingredient called CGF (Chlorella growth factor) derived from a hot water extract of the algae. It is estimated that tablets contain about 15% of chlorella growth factor.

The original discovery of this physiologically active substance was made in early 1950 by Dr. Fujimaki from the People's Scientific Research Centre Tokyo, Japan. Experiments have shown that CGF enhances RNA/DNA functions that are responsible for the pro-duction of proteins, enzymes and energy at the cellular level, and accelerates the growth and development of new cells in chlorella organisms.
This active substance is unique and only produced in the process of rapid multiplication through photo-synthesis.
The structure of CGF is quite complex. CGF consists mostly of a nuclear derivatives and a combination of water-soluble substances in the algae.
    It consists also of amino acids, sulfur, manganese, vitamins, polysaccharides, peptides (as glutathione) proteins and nucleic acid-coated substances as adenosine and cysteine nuclei, RNA DNA.

In human, there is the largest concentration of manganese in the skeletal, liver, pancreas and pituitary gland (the main gland of the endocrine system).

Manganese is fundamental and because of the lack of manganese, memory loss occurs in connection with aging. Manganese is needed for metabolism of protein, carbohydrates and liver and can play an important role in the formation of blood.

Manganese is also important for the nervous system, the brain and for the production of sex hormones as well as for the skeleton. You should not underestimate the importance of manganese for the body's chemistry and metabolism. The nuclei of CGF contains the six sugars glucose, mannose, rhamnose, arabinose, galactose, and xylose.

The peptide's amino acid structure contains glutamic acid, aspartic acid, alanine, serine, glycine and proline. Polysaccharides were the first substances that were isolated and examined from chlorella extract (CGF). One of these also contains sulfur. Chlon A, as the Japanese called it, could show anti-inflammatory and anti-tumor results.

In separate experiments, it was disclosed that Chlon A prevented growth of tumor cells. The researchers believe that Chlon A really is a beta glucan.
(An acidic polysaccharide Chlon A from Chlorella pyrenoidosa physiochemical and biological properties, Chemotherapy (Japan) 1982; 30(9):pp. 1041-1046).
(An acidic polysaccharide Chlon A from Chlorella pyrenoidosa.
Anti-tumor activity and immunological response, Chemotherapy Japan 1986; 34(4):pp. 302-307).

If you eat 1 gram of chlorella by every meal (5 x 200 mg) the content of proteins is only 667 mg but it contains 29,5 mg RNA and 2,8 mg DNA which helps to protect cells and increase your energy level.

Dr. Benjamin Frank (the "first" doctor) pointed to RNA as the first anti-aging factor. As author of the book "The No-Ageing Diet," he pointed out that human RNA / DNA production progressively slows down with age, resulting in lower levels of vitality and increased susceptibility to various diseases. He therefore recommended a high intake of food rich in nucleic acids. Nucleic acids are important for survival because they are in the cells.

These nucleic acids control the reproduction of new cells, cell division, cell growth and energy production. Polysaccharides are effective in stimulating the immune system. For long, it has been considered that sardines in oil contain the most RNA. Recently, it has been found that chlorella pyrenoidosa contains about 17 times more RNA than sardines.
Researchers have discovered that CGF is produced by chlorella during intense photosynthesis that allows chlorella to grow rapidly.

A cell divides into four new cells every 20 - 24 hours and CGF supports this rapid rate of reproduction. Chlorella Growth Factor (CGF) promotes growth in animals and microorganisms and renews our cells. Experiments with microorganisms in children and animals have shown that CGF promotes faster growth than normal without reversing side effects. In adults, CGF appears to enhance the functions of RNA DNA responsible for the production of proteins, enzymes and energy at the cellular level, promoting tissue repair and acting as the protection of cells against a variety of toxic substances. CGF strengthens the growth of the friendly lactobacillus in the intestine by up to 400% according to researchers. CGF fixes damaged tissues and protects cells from toxic substances in children and adults.

CGF does not stimulate growth or contribute to weight gain in adults, nor is it known that CGF can stimulate the growth of any disease. CGF only stimulates growth in children and animals that have not yet achieved their full development. These results (increased selective growth and healing) can not be explained to be responsible for any other component of Chlorella than its unique growth factor (CGF).

Many researchers, academics and doctors around the world are currently in the process of learning how CGF works. Researchers report that CGF is produced during the most intense periods of photosynthesis, including the healing energy of the sunlight within its structure, (Drucker).

In a hospital, chlorella growth factor was used in patients with prolonged ulcers (gastric ulcer and chronic gastritis) who refused to heal during treatment with common drugs.

For patients who received CGF, new tissues occurred shortly and all became quickly and completely healthy. This clearly shows that CGF was able to stimulate the healing of tissues when their own body tissues were exhausted. (Jensen).

Dr. Bernard Jensen wrote in his book. **Chlorella, Gem of the Orient**, that CGF and nucleic acids are the most valuable substances in chlorella because they raise the total energy level in the body as a whole and repair and renew all body organs, glands and tissues. CGF is the most valuable substance in chlorella and is found exclusively in chlorella which may be a contributing factor to this algae plant being the most popular nutritional supplement in Japan today.

Chlorella and the detoxification process

Chlorella is a powerful aid to the body's remediation of heavy metals and other pesticides. By detoxification, it is meant to eliminate toxic substances from the body. This is a natural process that the body must constantly undergo when exposed to toxic chemicals, pesticides, drugs, heavy metals or other toxins produced in the body such as in the intestine caused by ineffective metabolism.

Methods of detoxification

Poisons have different decomposition rates and depending on this and how much amount of poison is added, the damage may be acute and most difficult to remove are fat-soluble, non-polar substances.

There are different methods of disposal, such as water and juice fasting, that can sometimes cause more harm than good.

A study was carried out in 2002 by Dr. Silva and colleagues who found that low doses of phytochemicals in chlorella can support the functions of the body's detoxification process. According to scientific studies, chlorella has a highly effective ability to remove heavy metals, not least mercury.

Chlorella cell nucleus is surrounded by a cell wall of three layers of which the middle one consists of cellulose micro fibers.

This is a carotene-like material that contains the subtle *sporopollenin* (a naturally occurring carotene) that is resistant to degradation and capable of attracting heavy metals as well as body extraneous bacteria.

Using chlorophyll and fractions of chlorella's strong cell wall, these heavy metals and other toxins are then carried out through the intestinal tract.

On their way out of the body systems, these aids seek to clear intestinal walls from plaque and bowel pockets from existing waste, then bring the toxins out of the bowel. Of course, it is important to have at least one or more bowel movement each day to help the body to more effectively be eliminated of toxins of different kinds.

Here too, chlorella plays its important role in strengthening our own lactic acid bacteria so that they, in turn, can work more efficiently to maintain a good intestinal balance and thereby streamline our bowel movements.

In Japan, the interest in chlorella is focused on its detoxifying properties and in its ability to neutralize or re-move toxic substances from the body. Japan has previously experienced the effects of nuclear by-products in the most catastrophic way.

The penalty was growing problems with industrial environmental damage such as disease of Mini-Mata.

People began then to be interested in the fight against environmental hazards considerably more.

People around the world have long been familiar with medical reports on chlorella's properties to effectively contribute to detoxification of both environment and human. Another Japanese study on heavy metal poisoning revealed that when 8 grams of chlorella were allocated daily to experimental animals, secretion increased threefold of cadmium and dioxin at the intestinal discharge and sevenfold of the urine.

Also in the United States, long time studies have shown chlorella's detoxification ability in animal and human experiments. Already in 1950, it was found that chlorella also had the ability to increase the resistance to harmful X-rays due to its large contents of chlorophyll. The American Army found the same thing when they made a study.

Poison-absorbing properties inherent in the structure of chlorella's cell wall.
Chlorella pyrenoidosa has a distinct cell wall structure with a chemical composition that is partly responsible for algae detoxification ability.

Pore RS, 1984. Detoxification of chlordecone poisoned rats with chlorella and chlorella derived sporopollenin. Drug-Chem Toxic 7(11.57-71)

The cell wall consists of about 31% hemicellulose, 27% protein, 15% alpha cellulose, 9.2% lipids, 5.2% ash and 3.3% glucosamine.

Northcote OH et al., 1958. The chemical composition and structure of the cell wall of Chlorella pyrenoidosa. Biohem.J 70.391-97

Scientific research shows that the cell wall of the algae contains constellations (most likely cellulose and polysaccharide that adhere to and remove heavy metals such as cadmium, lead and mercury from the body.

Jensen B. 1987. Chlorella: Gem of the Orient. Bernard Jensen Publisher, Escondido, CA, USA and Travieso RO et al. 1999. Heavy Metal Removal by Micro-algae. Bull. Environ Contain. Toxicol. 62: 144-151

Similarly, research has shown that the cell wall whose active ingredients that contribute to detoxification, remain intact despite that the cell wall is being powdered, yet accelerates removal of hazardous chlorinated hydrocarbons insecticides from the body.
(Pore RS. 1984. Detoxification of chlordecone poisoned rats with chlorella and chlorella derived sporopollenin. Drug-Chem-Toxicol 7(11.57-711)

Chlorella works to remove toxins from the body such as heavy metals, poisons and foreign body bacteria. This activation help us to eliminate dioxins and other hormone disturbing substances.
Chlorella is the richest natural source of chlorophyll, which is a powerful cleaner and detoxifier, and is the content of the strong cell wall of special fibre that bind to and afterwards remove an amount of unwanted toxins from the body.

This activity helps to free the burden of the liver, assist it and strengthen it so that it can work more efficiently.
A large amount of research results in USA and Europe show that chlorella can assist the body to eliminate stubborn hydrocarbons and heavy metals such as mercury, cadmium and lead, DDT and PCB while strengthening our immune system.

In Japan, interest in chlorella has been focused on its detoxifying properties and its ability to clear or neutralize toxic substances from the body. It is the powerful fibre-like material in chlorella that enhances bowel capacity and improves our bowel movements.

Good and regular bowel movement is a very important part of our own body's attempt to have a natural purification process.

You need to eat two to three meals of food a day, empty the bowel twice a day or every six hours. Most people suffer from constipation due to that they consume highly processed foods that do not contain enough fibers. Fibre is what causes good bowel movements and which also binds to heavy metals and other toxic substances and expels these from the body.

Bowel-cancer is the second most common type of cancer and may be caused by having used lots of highly processed food that lacks fibre. In areas in the world, where primitive substances are still being used, as in the African countryside, there is hardly any intestinal cancer. Researchers recommend that we daily should eat at least 25 to 30 grams of fibre to seek to prevent bowel cancer, and despite this, the average man consumes only about 11 grams per day.

A clean blood with a variety of red blood cells that transports oxygen is necessary to get a strong immune system.

Chlorella's cleansing activity of the intestine and other elimination channels, as well as its ability to protect and strengthen the liver, helps keep the blood clean.

Pure blood ensures that metabolic residues are removed from tissues.

The purification process is normal and important to the overall health of the body's various functions.

Doctor Ichimura at Toyama University gave 30 daily oral chlorine tablets (approximately 6 g) to 30 patients suffering from heavy metal poisoning.

He reported that heavy metals were removed from the body when emptying the intestines.

Our environment of chemicals and heavy metals is often affected and this report on chlorella is considered a remarkable scientific discovery. (Hagano Ichimura).

Important new study shows that Chlorella pyrenoidosa helps to reduce the exposure of dangerous chemicals to newborns.

Japanese researchers have recently published the result of a unique study, confirming that Chlorella pyrenoidosa has the ability to greatly reduce the transmission of the fatal poisons dioxins, furans and PCBs from mother to fetus.

Nakano, S; et al., maternal fetal distribution and transfer of dioxins in pregnant women in Japan, and attempts to reduce maternal transfer with Chlorella pyrenoidosa supplements: June 2005.

Besides from that pregnant mothers who ate Chlorella pyrenoidosa could prevent their fetuses from being exposed to these toxins in the uterus, it also appeared that their breast milk contained a significantly smaller amount of the toxins.

While a larger number of previous animal studies reported cholesterol's detoxifying capacity, relatively few studies have been found to have been able to document this ability in human trials.

Animal-based studies published in the 1980s and 1990s indicated that chlorella could delay the abolition of chlorinated hydrocarbon used in the production of a variety of agricultural chemicals such as, for example, pesticides.

Chlorella is used in many countries in the heavy metal detoxification process. Chlorella pyrenoidosa can rapidly excrete mercury, cadmium and other toxic metals without interfering with the balance of essential minerals, a problem associated with the use of synthetic chelating agents. Dioxins, and their closest chemical cousins known as furans, are extremely endangered environmental pollutants that are produced as byproducts to a large number of industrial processes, including chlorination, paper production and the production of all PVC products.

These poisons are produced, not only at the manufacturing stage, but are even released when the products are burned at the end of their life cycle.

A form of dioxin, known as 2.3.7.8-TCDD, is one of the most toxic chemicals known to man and is classified as Class1 cancerogeneic (known to cause cancer in humans).

The Japanese dioxin study provides us with convincing evidence that one of the easiest ways to protect us from harmful effects of toxic substances, is to eat a high quality supplement of chlorella pyrenoidosa every day. The latest study fully complements the importance of previous research with chlorella by confirming that this plant can effectively detoxify the body from any toxic element tested so far and that this option applies to both humans and animals.

It is crucial that you choose to use an additive of chlorella pyrenoidosa, cultivated under strictly sanitary conditions and tested for the absence of toxic substances in itself.

There are a number of family members of chlorella available today, but only chlorella pyrenoidosa contains the unique component known as sporopollenin which has been shown to play an important role in the process of chemical poisoning.

The latest evidence from Japan, taking into account the two latest reports from the Environmental Working Group, should help convince anyone interested in the good health of his own and his family, to place chlorella pyrenoidosa at the top of the list of supplement to be eaten every day.

Pore, RS. "Detoxification of chlordecone poisoned rats with Chlorella and chlorella derived sporopollenin. Drug Chem Toxicol. 198 7 (0: 57-71

Chlorella strengthens the immune system.

In 1908, the scientist Metchnikoff received the Nobel Prize because of his discoveries around the immune system.

Immunology or studies of our immune system is probably one of the most interesting and grateful areas of modern medicine research. Immunology is about development and the ability of the body's mechanisms being used to fight foreign invaders, whether they are bacteria, viruses, chemicals or foreign proteins.

The immune system is the front line of the body's own protection against disease, whether it is infection or degeneration.

When our immune system weakens, we become more susceptible to diseases from colds to more serious problems such as diabetes and cancer.

Many years of researches and experiences show that chlorella has a stimulating and potentiating effect on the immune system.

B-cells are active in fighting bacteria, T-cells are active against viruses and cancer and macrophages are active against different cancer diseases, foreign proteins and chemicals.

Macrophages are large cells that are located in tissues such as liver (Kuppfer cells), spleen, lymph nodes, thymus, lungs, abdomen, blood (monocytes), joints, bone marrow and connective tissues and actively they purify the blood, body fluids and cavities from harmful substances.

As there is a limited number of macrophages in a human body, they have only limited ability to expel harmful substances from the bloodstream.

One way to fight cancer is to use agents that stimulate both production and activity in macrophages. Stimulants of these contribute to increased destruction of cancer cells and also increase the removal of harmful cancer residues in the blood through its phagocytes.

Antibodies are large Y-shaped protein molecules whose primary task is to bind and distinguish foreign bodies in the body so that other parts of the immune system can recognize them and then break them down.

In each of the two shapes of the Y, the antibody has the anti-body surfaces that bind foreign matters.

The shaft contains signals that are recognized of other parts of the immune system.

When an anti-body is attached to a foreign substance, the following actions are taken: The shaft is recognized by a special type of macrophages called (big eater cels).

When a macrophage recognizes and binds to the shaft of an anti-body, it embraces that antibody and all that is bound to it in order to, in the first place, enclose the foreign matter and then to destroy it.

Interferon is a natural protein in the body and is considered to make a physiological stimulus for macrophages.

When hot water extracts of chlorella (CGF) were infected in mice, it was observed that high levels of interferon were spotted in the blood, already 2.5 hours after the injection. The first experiment with chlorella ability to stimulate the formation of interferon in the body was performed in 1973 by Dr. Kojima and his co-workers.

Further studies with chlorella showed unidentified serum factors that were also involved in stimulating macrophages. From the early 70's, many studies have shown that chlorella enhances the immune system through its ability to stimulate macrophages.

T-cells and defense against viruses.

In order to defend themselves against virus attacks, antibodies and macrophages are not enough.

Virus or cellular parasites enter the cells, use them to copy themselves as much as possible and then send them further into the body to hide and to infect new cells. In the new cell, the virus copies itself as before and is considered in its hidden state to be more dangerous than as a free virus particle. In order to provide an effective protection that can defend us from viruses, the immune system now needs to kill the cells that are infected by the virus itself.

The body can, without danger, lose some of its cells, as it is created new ones by dividing adjacent cells. The immune system uses special killer cells that have the primary and only task of searching, recognizing and killing virus-infected cells. It is now considered that these killer cells wander around the body and feel one cell after another.

Since they find a cell that contains the virus, they hold the cell for less than a quarter, kill it and then continue looking for new ones. These killer cells are also called T-cells and use a protein called T-cell receptor to select their victims. The body's natural defense system is based on mutual support from all organs, glands, tissues and body function. In order to maintain strong defense against diseases, we should avoid breaking down the body itself.

Our best defense against diseases is a clean, strong body with a proper chemical balance in our tissues. If we allow our tissues to be burdened by cataracts, chemical additives in the food, excessive and in many cases unnecessary intake of drugs, smoking, sprinkled fruits and vegetables and other foods, chemicals in contaminated air, treated drinking water, substances that the body can not afford, our tissues become ineffective to the extent that they become an easy change for chronic diseases.

It can be noted that the strength of our natural defense system depends on how well we take care of our genetically inherited weaknesses, how we maintain the correct mineral density in the tissues, how to avoid toxic body build-up and how we prevent the under-activity of our tissues. These factors are almost always interconnected. If the tissue is under-active, it is usually toxically charged. If it is toxic, it generally takes one or more minerals to make this tissue function normally. If the tissue lacks one or more minerals, it is usually a hereditary weak tissue which has been wrongly nourished or has been exposed to excessive stress or over efforts.

If the body is not strong, the hereditary weakening tissues are usually toxic due to a toxic charged blood flow.

If blood and lymph are not clean, the intestine is not clean and is not very active in order to be emptied quickly enough. The body's detoxifying organs as intestine, lungs and bronchus, skin protection, kidneys and skin should be active. Their primary task is to detoxify the body from residues that otherwise lead to toxic load.

Some of the latest scientific experiments in Japan and the Republic of China deal with chlorella's effects on the immune system in the event of degenerative diseases. Many years ago, Japanese doctors discovered that when they gave chlorella to cancer patients under-going radiation therapy or chemotherapy, these patients avoided a rapid drop in white blood cells.

The consequences of a rapid drop in the white blood cells can be characterized by fatigue, low energy levels, weak resistance and other degrading conditions.

Doctors found that when chlorella was given **prior** to the above treatment methods, one could avoid the value of the white blood cells to be falling too deeply.

In addition, a faster return to a more normalized blood value was found in patients treated with chlorella before and during cancer treatment.

Researchers at Kitazato Institute indicated that chemical substances in chlorella stimulated the production of interferon, a protein in the body which protects cells against viruses and is considered to slow down the growth of cancer cells.

Interferon is one of the most important natural defenses against cancer. One way to fight cancer is to
use substances that can stimulate the production of
macrophages and their activity.

Interferon is a natural secretion in the body that is
considered to be the stimulus of macrophages and
tumor-necrotic factor (TNF).
Chlorella stimulates the activity of T-cells and macrophages by raising the level of interferon and thereby
enhancing the immune system's ability to fight foreign
invaders, whether it be bacteria, virus, chemicals or
foreign proteins.
It has been suggested that chlorella's unique cell wall
contains complex polysaccharides which contribute to
increased interferon production, which can strengthen
the ability to fight cancer cells.
Chlorella's unique cell wall is therefore one of the most
important factors that differ significantly from other
green foods. When hot extracts of chlorella were injected into mice, high doses of interferon were
observed in the blood already 2.5 hours after injection.
It was found that activity of extract from chlorella
occurred 72 hours after injection and that the stimulatory effect decreased slowly after two weeks.

The material used in these experiments was found
to have a molecular weight of 1250, be water soluble
and completely free of toxins.
Upon examination of the mice tissues, it was shown
that the macrophages had increased activity.
To confirm this in another study, macrophages were
taken from the abdomen on rats recently injected with
chlorella extracts and examined under microscopy.

These macrophages proved much more active in
absorbing carbon particles than in the control group,

which shows that macrophagocyte (macrophage's swelling of microorganisms) had occurred.

Further studies found unidentifiable serum factors that were also involved in stimulating the immune system by stimulating macrophages (Rei Bunso, Health Revolution, Nisshosha Co. Lid., Kyoto, Japan).

Chlorella stimulates the immune factors.
Science believes that trillions of white blood cells (leukocytes) circulating in the blood and lymph is the body's main defense system against disease. Leukocytes of similar types not only circulate, but gather in lymph nodes and lymphatic tissues such as tonsils myeloma and appendicitis. They wear the walls of the liver passages, where they are known as *kupfer cells* and in parts of the small intestine.
Interferon thus protects cells from harmful viruses. Interferon is a natural secretion in the body and is considered a physiological stimulator of macrophages.
    The defenders of these immune systems have the task of patrolling the blood and lymph or standing on guard in the lymph nodes, living the intestine, the mile etc. and break down harmful bacteria, remove foreign substances as well as fora old blood cells out of circulation. The cells and antibodies of the immune system can be destroyed by radiation and chemo-therapy. Research has shown that a significant loss of white blood cells occurs two times in tanning because the white blood cells moving through the skin's capillaries are destroyed by the ultraviolet light from the sun.
    White blood cell (leukocytes) and antibodies demand both a good nutrition balance and high quality

proteins. If we do not eat properly, the immune system and other parts of the body are damaged. **Chlorella is an excellent stimulus for the immune system, which is one of chlorella's most prominent benefits.**

Chlorella is well-known in Japanese science community as a biological response modifier which implies a natural substance that enhances the capacity of the body's own immune system.
Scientific studies have confirmed that chlorella may supply all important nutrients to individuals with impaired immune systems, especially when they are exposed to stress.

At an immunology conference in France in 1985, it was reported that research that showed how stimulation of the immune system, could counteract tumors.
In summary, researchers found that chlorella could enhance activity for macrophages and that some lymphocytes were capable of breaking down cells.
It was checked whether the registered anti-tumor effect could be a synergistic effect of activated macrophages and toxic T-cells. However, it was considered that the anti-tumor effect is mainly due to strong macrophage activity.

Chlorella is 10% RNA (ribonucleic acid) and 3% DNA (deoxyribonucleic acid) and CGF has a concentration of these complicated macromolecules.
Chlorella has the highest amount of nucleotides among known foods. RNA and DNA are nuclear factors whose reproduction occurs naturally in our body and decreases with age, perhaps already from the age of 20. Dr. Bernard Jensen, one of the world's most knowledgeable and reputable nutritionists, emphasis

the importance of daily use of a diet rich in these macromolecules.

As humans age, the cellular process becomes slower. The cell wall that regulates fluid, nutritional intake and bowel function becomes less functional As a result, nutrient uptake is effective and more poisonous waste remains in the cells.

This, in turn, leads to increased acidification in the body as favoring many types of chronic and degrading diseases.

As we have a satisfactory intake of food, rich in RNA and DNA that can defend our own macro-molecules, the cell wall continues to function efficiently by keeping the clue clean and supply it with nutrients.

If our RNA and DNA are in good condition and therefore able to function effectively, we can better absorb nutrients, get rid of poisons and avoid many diseases, the cells will be able to repair themselves and the body's energy levels and vitality increases. An intake of chlorella by each meal, a total of 3 grams per day, gives us 390 mg of RNA and DNA, an in-valuable aid in repairing and restoring our cells.

If we wish to help our body to self-healing and even ward off our disease, it is necessary to strengthen our own immune system.

Most viral infections and pathogenic attacks can be fought successfully if the cells are healthy and if the metabolic tissues are clean and clear. A strong immune system keeps pathogen in check and wards disease away.

Beta-glucans are polysaccharides that occur in big amounts in some of today's most fascinating and powerful medicinal foods such as the healing fungi, reishi and shiitake, as well as in micro-algae like chlor-ella. Beta-glucans have been shown to be strong stimulators of the immune system. It is thought that they accelerate the release of powerful chemicals that activate the immune cells. The macrophages actually have a specific receptor layer for beta-glucans as a kind of *lock and key mechanism* that activates their immune cells.

It is suspected that beta-glucans can be the key nu-tritions that give the possibilities for substances to act "biological responders" which enhance immune function and produce anti-tumor influences.

Glycoproteins are protein-carbohydrate complexes. A number of glycoproteins filtered from chlorella has been shown to stimulate the activity of immune cells targeting cells invaded by viruses or cancer.

A water soluble anti-tumor glycoprotein from chlorella, Planta Medica, 1996: 62nd pp. 123-12)

Protective effect of an acidic glycoprotein obtained from culture of chlorella against myelosuppression by 5-fluorouracil, Cancer Immunology Immunotherapy, June 1996: 42 pp. 268 741).

A unique glycoprotein isolated from Chlorella not only stimulated T-cell activity but also helped to mobilize them against the tumor's location. The results were so clear, that the researchers suggested that treatment with this substance before surgery could prevent the spread of tumors to other sites as well as their further progress.

(Novel glycoprotein obtained from Chlorella strain CK22 shows anti metastatic immune potential. Immunotherapy, 1998:4:pp.313-20)

Chlorella promotes healthy cellular growth and repair, which can delay aging.

All of the above mentioned properties of chlorella work together to promote the body's own ability, to heal, which means a longer and healthier life. This is what makes chlorella effective against the problems caused by a modern and often incorrect lifestyle.
All of the above mentioned activities with chlorella can help us to prevent illness and disease.

Our cells are renewed continuously.
Given the correct nutritional support of GGF and RNA/ DNA, it is not surprising that we are beneficially affected by chlorella. With the help of these compounds in chlorella, the similar effects of the body become more profound. Scientific studies show chlorella's resources and the ability to alleviate specific health problems such as hypertension, diabetes, malignant tumors, fibromyalgia and others.
However, chlorella is a naturally produced food, not a drug produced and added to it by human.

Consuming chlorella in order to strengthen the immune system is fundamentally different from using a medication for treating disease.
Pharmaceutical drugs are mainly designed for symptom treatment. They are not meant to be able to treat the underlying problem that causes symptoms.
Because the original problem persists, symptoms continues. Even worse is that long-term consumption of strong drugs can usually lead to side effects for the patient.

We all need to take care of our health.
Perhaps, more than ever, one should consider which way to promote one's immune system in order to avoid getting sick. Act on the problems in the opposite

direction as they turn out be. To use a true and healthy diet is the key to preventive medication.
In addition, it is important to detoxify the body every day from foreign bacteria and heavy metals found in air, water and food.

What is good to eat?
Feed containing enough fiber.
Food that does not contain too much refined carbohydrates and other refined foods.
Food that does not contain trans-fats from refined fat (fried foods, margarine and others).
Food containing more essential fatty acids like omega-3 and instead less of omega-6.
Food which has a variety of vitamins, minerals, phytochemicals, acids and enzymes.

Chlorella stimulates digestion
Chlorella contributes to intestinal cleansing and generally better bowel health by activating effective peristaltic. In regular contractions, the intestinal wall muscles are affected in such a way that the intestinal contents are kept in motion.
This process prevents constipation and contributes to prevent the return of toxic material from the stool to the bloodstream. Smelly stools are largely avoided by shortening the decay process due to better, more efficient combustion and elimination of poisons.
Chlorella contains a variety of components that are helpful to our digestive system; enzymes, fiber and the high chlorophyll content are attributed to the possibility that help people to eliminate bad breath after a couple of days. Chlorella also helps to propagate and at the same time, enhance the effect of friendly lactic acid bacteria in the intestine, which

improves digestion and absorption of nutrition in the blood flow.

These lactic acid bacteria (lactobacteria), also help prevent the growth of pathogens commonly found in the intestinal tract, such as Candida albicans (sometimes called yeast infection)
In addition, preventing constipation, the good intestinal flora, stimulated by chlorella, helps to combat infections.
It also helps to neutralize any toxic substances in the diet and also produces some important vitamin B12. Fractions of the non-digestible part of chlorella's cell wall, (about 20%) act as fiber in the intestine and stimulate peristalsis. Chlorella contains enzymes such as chlorophyllis and pepsin as well as digestive enzymes, that perform a number of important and health promoting functions in the body.

Chlorella normalizes blood sugar.
(Lee HT et al., Hypoglycemic Action of Chlorella. "Journal of the Formosan Medical Association, Vol. 76, No. 3, March 1977, pp. 272-276).

Experiments performed show that chlorella appears to be able to normalize too low blood sugar while personal testimony shows that so is also the case with diabetes (high blood sugar).
Having a normal level of blood sugar is essential for having a normal brain function, cardiac function and energy metabolism, all of which are crucial for maintaining good health and assist yourself to prevent diseases.
The liver and pancreas are busy to regulate blood sugar. We find that chlorella supports and balances the

abdominal pain function, strengthens the liver as well as other organs we talked about.

In addition, vitamins and minerals which affect sugar metabolism such as zinc, potassium and magnesium are recommended.

These substances are found in completely 100% organic and natural form in chlorella. The sugar metabolism is controlled by vitamins and trace elements. In the case of shortages, you often feel a need for the missing vitamins and minerals. If the biological balance is not restored, sugar incineration can break down and type 2 diabetes or age diabetes can develop.

......**and blood pressure**.

Dental root problems in the 4th and 5th teeth of the upper jaw can contribute too high blood pressure. Hypertension is one of the major risk factors for heart attacks and strokes which are attributed to more deaths than any other disease. Laboratory tests have shown that regular use of Chlorella lowers high blood pressure and prevents stroke risk.

Low blood pressure is good if not due to a weak heart. People with lower blood pressure are often much more sensitive to side effects of medicines.

One may feel like fainting or feeling sick. It is therefore important to refrain from medication as much as possible if you have low blood pressure.

(Murakami, T. The influence of Chlorella as a Food Supplement on High Blood Pressure and as Stroke Preventative for Rats ", Shouva 58-nen Nibon nogica gakkai Koen Yoshi 1983.)

For many years, it has been found in many documented cases, that Chlorella can normalize blood pressure.
High blood pressure is the main risk factor for myocardial infarction and stroke, which can be attributed to the biggest cause of death of all diseases in the world. Laboratory trials with rats have also shown that regular use of chlorella lowers too high blood pressure and prevent strokes attacks.
The number of cases of low blood pressure is fewer, and when using Chlorella during month-long periods, blood pressure har risen to the normal level.

Chlorella stimulates production of albumin.
Japanese researchers recently discovered that chlorella can raise blood levels of albumin.
Albumin is one of the body's most powerful antioxidants as well as an important transport system through the body for vitamins, minerals, fatty acids, hormones and other essential substances.
Albumin is also active to remove toxins from cells to the liver where they break down and later are expelled from the body. Without adequate levels of albumin, the kidneys and other vital organs can not perform their work and the immune system can not function properly.
A number of studies have shown that low levels of albumin are a marker of serious diseases such as cancer and cardiovascular disease.

This was also confirmed by a British study, published in *The Lancet.* Over 7000 middle-aged men were followed up for 9 years.

The study showed that men with the lowest level of serum albumin had the highest death rate for various reasons including heart disease.

Our level of albumin is decreasing steadily as we age, which is another indication showing that albumin plays an important role in trying to keep our bodies healthy, strong and youthful. Albumin levels are usually lower in smokers.

Chlorella is beneficial in ulcerative colitis, fibromyalgia and other chronic health problems.

Researchers at Virginia Commonwealth University, Medical College of Virginia, Richmond, USA found promising results when using chlorella to treat chronic health problems such as ulcerative colitis and fibromyalgia.

They demonstrated on Chlorella's ability to alleviate symptoms, improve quality of life and normalize body functions in patients with fibromyalgia or ulcerative colitis. These effects can be attributed to a generally elevated immune function. (Merchant).

Animal experiments have also shown chlorella's protective properties in stress-related stomach ulcers.
    Chlorella is considered to prevent the formation of gastric ulcer mainly through immune enhancement and provide protection of the stomach/intestinal bacteria such as lactic acid bacteria.

Fatigue syndrome
Prolonged fatigue, fever, joint pain and depression are common symptoms in this chronic condition.

Stimulants and support for the immune system and adrenal glands are the most effective therapies. The adrenal glands can nourish the vitamins C, B complex and zinc, all of which can be added through chlorella.
A large number of people report the benefits of using chlorella in chronic fatigue syndrome as you get increased energy levels and decreased symptoms.

Chlorella has rejuvenating properties.
Chlorella contains not only powerful antioxidants but also an amount of nucleic acids, RNA and DNA which are predominantly in chlorella growth factor (CGF). RNA and DNA are the reproductive (genetic) substances present in each cell that vitalize cellular activity.
One often refers to *life extracts* that can delay the process of aging. Cells can repair themselves and the body's energy levels and vitality rise.
        Degradation of DNA and RNA in the cells is considered to be one of the main factors in aging and a risk of having degenerative diseases. (Frank)
Nucleic acids in digestion and assimilation are degraded and linked to other nutrients like vitamin B12, peptides and polysaccharides. This means that DNA and RNA which we eat directly, can not replace human cellular DNA and RNA, but provide us with their composition of amino acids after digestion and assimilation and provide us with building blocks for the repair of our genetic material.
    As man ages, the cellular process slows down. The cell wall that regulates liquids, nutrient uptake and waste disposal become less efficient. Nutritional intake becomes less effective and more toxic waste remains in the cells. This leads to increased acidity in the body that favors various types of chronic and degenerative diseases.

If we are having a satisfactory intake of foods rich in DNA and RNA to protect our own cellular nucleic acids, the cell wall continues to function effectively, keeping the cell clean and providing it with nutrition.

It is therefore important to eat chlorella regularly. RNA and DNA in chlorella are an invaluable aid for cellular repair and restoration.

Chlorella protects our health by providing support to cell-level functions to keep our bodies in good shape. Brew yeast is known to be a good source of RNA, but sardines in oil contain 10 times more than brew yeast (343 mg per 100 grams). Chlorella, however, supplies us with 10 times more RNA than sardines; 3000 mg per 100 grams!

Chlorella helps to normalize acid/base balances.

Our diet has been radically changed over the last eighty years. We do not eat enough vegetables and fruits in general which in turn, make up alkaline foods. Instead, we acidify our body system through fast food and other low-enzyme food. Either one has cooked or pasteurized or otherwise processed enzymes from the diet. Without enzymes, our body can not absorb important nutrients. What makes the situation even worse is that junk food creates an acidified environment in our body that will eventually provide an ideal environment for disease. For example **cancer does not endure in an alkaline environment, but thrives in acidified environment.**

What we consume either raises or lowers our pH which should be between 7.2-7.4 pH. As an example, soft drinks such as Coca Cola have a pH of 2.7-3.0 which is supersaturated. A soda with a pH of 3.0 gets a significantly higher pH after having passed through the

body; It will reach a pH of about 7.0 by stealing important minerals from the body.
By consuming soda and other acidifying foods, the body's pH value decreases and makes it more acidified and thus more possible for providing different diseases. The largest amount of cancer patients appears to have low pH, from 6.0 6.5 or lower.
The body simply can not fight disease if the pH value is not in the right balance. Therefore, increase the consumption of alkaline foods and reduce substances that can cause acidification in the body. Chlorella is rich in minerals, which the body uses as a buffer for acidification. Chlorella is an alkaline food!

Pregnancy
Japanese researchers have recently published the results of a unique study that confirms that Chlorella pyrenoidosa has the ability to greatly reduce the transmission of the deadly poisons dioxins, furans and PCBs from mother to fetus.
Nakano, S et al "Maternal-fetal distribution and transfer of dioxin pregnant women in Japan, and attempts to reduce maternal transfer with Chlorella (Chlorella pyrenoidosa) supplements." Chemosphere: June 2005

This result suggests that supplementation of Chlorella, significantly reduces the risk of pregnancy associated anaemia, proteinuria and edema. Chlorella supplement may be useful as a resource of natural folate, vitamin B-12 and iron for pregnant women.
Results of a present study confirm that the quantity of dioxins transferred to fetuses is closely correlated to dioxin concentrations in maternal adipose tissue or, cumulative quantities of dioxins in the body.

The latent risks of environmental contaminants such as dioxins may well be appearing in the form of symptoms such as ADHD and LD in children, who are more sensitive than adults to chemical substances and toxins.

A study looking at mother's breastfeeding found that those taking chlorella had increased levels of IgA, the body's natural defense antibodies that can help protect babies. Chlorella pyrenoidosa helped clear dioxin, a toxin, from the milk [Source: Nakano].

In addition to meeting nutritional requirements, breast milk plays important roles in biodefense for nursing infants. Dioxins have been detected at high concentrations in breast milk, raising concerns about disorders in nursing infants caused by breast milk containing dioxins in Japan.
We analyzed dioxin levels in breast milk and maternal blood samples from 35 pregnant women in Japan.
        We also measured immunoglobulin IgA concentrations in breast milk and investigated correlations with dioxin concentrations.
In addition, 18 of the 35 women took Chlorella pyrenoidosa supplements during pregnancy, and the effects on dioxin and IgA concentrations in breast milk were investigated.
Toxic equivalents were significantly lower in the breast milk of women taking Chlorella tablets than in the Control group (P = .003).
One human study has been conducted with 6 g Chlorella during pregnancy from gestational week 12-18 (variable start date) until delivery, and was generally well tolerated with no reported adverse effects on mother or apparent adverse effects on off-spring.

Interestingly, toxicological reports indicate that Chlorella is associated with less leg edema (water retention and swelling) at 6g daily relative to control with 44.7% of women in control reporting leg edema in the third trimester, yet only 9.4% reporting edema with 6g Chlorella.

One study in pregnant women noted that 6g of Chlorella were associated with less urinary proteins, suggesting protective effect mechanisms unknown.

IMPORTANT NEW STUDY SHOWS THAT CHLORELLA PYRENOIDOSA CONTRIBUTES TO A REDUCTION OF NEW-BORNED BABIE'S EXPOSURE TO DANGEROUS CHEMICAL TOXINS.

When pregnant mothers who were eating chlorella pyrenoidosa could prevent their fetuses to be exposed to these toxins, it was also found that their breast milk contained significantly smaller or no amount of toxins.

While a greater number of previous animal studies reported chlorella's detoxifying capacity, there have been relatively few studies have been able to document this ability in human trials.

Animal-based studies published during the 1980s and 1990s indicated that chlorella could speed up the removal of chlorinated hydrocarbon used in the manufactures of a variety of agricultural chemicals such as pesticides.

Chlorella pyrenoidosa (Chlorella) supplements during pregnancy, and the effects on dioxin and IgA concentrations in breast milk were investigated. Toxic equivalents were significantly lower in the breast milk of women taking Chlorella tablets than in the Control group (P = .003).

These results suggest that Chlorella supplementation by the mother may reduce transfer of dioxins to the child through breast milk.

Chlorella is used in many countries in the detoxification process of heavy metals.
Chlorella pyrenoidosa can speed up excretion of mercury, cadmium and other toxic metals without disturbing the balance of essential minerals.
This is otherwise a problem linked to the use of the synthetic chelating agents.

Dioxins and their closest chemical cousins, known, as furans are extremely persistent to environmental pollutants, produced as by-products to a large number of industrial processes that include chlorination, including paper and the production of all products with PVC.
These toxins are produced not only by the production stages, but released even when the products are burned up at the end of their life cycle.

One form of dioxin, known as TCDD 2,37,8, is one of the most toxic chemicals, known to man and is classified as Class 1 carcinogen (known to cause cancer in human).
Japanese studies of dioxins are showing that the best way to save you from it, is to eat a good quality of chlorella pyrenoidosa every day.
As there are several different "family members" of the chlorella family, it is most interesting that only chlorella pyrenoidosa is containing **sporopollenin**, which is capable of a more efficient detoxification process in the body.
This is why I also would like to advice pregnant becoming women, already in good time before pregnancy, to eat chlorella pyrenoidosa every day.

This is because it is of the most important matter to be able to give birth to a healthy human being.

These results suggest that supplementation of Chlorella to the mother may reduce transfer dioxins to the child through breast milk.

No significant correlation was identified between dioxin and IgA concentrations in breast milk in the Control group.

This, unfortunately, stresses the need for nutrients like this to keep our detoxification systems strong since nearly all of the women tested in the study had some level of dioxin.

It is unlikely that normal levels of dioxin exposure via food have a remarkable influence on IgA in breast milk

IgA concentrations in breast milk in Chlorella group were significantly higher than in the Control group ($P=.03$).

Increasing IgA levels in breast milk is considered to be effective for reducing the risk of infection in nursing infants.

The present results suggest that Chlorella supplementation not only reduces dioxin levels in breast milk, but may also have beneficial effects on nursing infants by increasing IgA levels in breast milk.

Nowadays it's usually a happy moment when a person becomes pregnant. Even happier is it if the mother is healthy and feels in good shape.

Folic acid, or vitamin B9 helps build healthy cells.

The body's need for folic acid increases during periods of rapid growth such as pregnancy and fetal development.

References:

Shiro Nakano Saiseikai Nara Hospital, Nara, Hokkaido, Japan.

Hideo Takekoshi Department of Bio resource Science, Obihiro University of Agriculture and Veterinary Medicine, Hokkaido, Japan Hokkaido Medicinal Plant Research Institute, Hokkaido, Japan.

Masuo Nakano Department of Bio resource Science, Obihiro University of Agriculture and Veterinary Medicine, Hokkaido, JapanHokkaido Medicinal Plant Research Institute, Hokkaido, Japan Rakuno Gakuen University, Hokkaido, Japan.

Research shows that women who become pregnant should consume a multivitamin with folic acid, which can reduce the risk of spina bifida occult by about 70%. Chlorella contains abundant protein and chlorophyll compared with other plants and also has large quantities of minerals such as iron and magnesium and vitamins, foliates, vitamin B6 and vitamin B12.
The proteins of Chlorella contain all the essential amino acids required for human growth and health.
    Chlorella and its extracts have been reported to exert a variety of effects including lowering of serum cholesterol and anti tumor activity.
In addition, several studies have demonstrated that Chlorella intake improved iron deficiency anaemia in rats, and suppressed elevation of blood pressure in rat models or human subjects.
    Thus, the aim of this study is to evaluate the preventive effects of Chlorella supplement, which is

rich in vitamins and minerals, on pregnancy anaemia in pregnant women.
The results of this study suggested that Chlorella supplementation significantly reduces the risk of pregnancy associated anaemia, proteinuria and edema.
Furthermore Chlorella supplement was well tolerated and no side effect was observed.

In conclusion, the consumption of Chlorella supplement was found to result in the significant reduction of the risk of anaemia, proteinuria and edema in pregnant women.
It appears that the beneficial effects of Chlorella pyrenoidosa supplement for pregnant women are due to the synergistic contribution of micronutrients in chlorella pyrenoidosa and the Influence on the immune system.
        Chlorella pyrenoidosa supplement is likely to be useful not only to pregnant women but to the large population with deficiency of iron or foliate as well.
It is essential for pregnant women to avoid heavy metals to be transmitted to the fetus. Previous research indicates that fetal and childhood exposure to toxic metals and deficiencies of nutritional elements are linked with several adverse developmental outcomes including intellectual disability and language, attention, and behavioral problems.
        Exposure to certain heavy metal toxins as well as impaired up-take of some essential minerals during late pregnancy and in the early postnatal period, are also triggers for the disorder.
To identify specific environmental exposures that increase autism risk, researchers gathered evidence from baby teeth.

For example, children are particularly susceptible to the effects of lead because their nervous systems are still developing.

A high percentage of children under the age of five have toxic levels of this heavy metal in their blood.

Anxious parents in the world have been waiting a long time to get definitive answers about the causes of Autism Spectrum Disorder (ASD).

An AD, which now affects one in 68 children, causes serious behavioral, social and communication issues.

A healthy baby.

Nowadays, it's usually a happy moment when you get pregnant. A happier thing is if the prospective mother is healthy and feeling in good shape. However, if the condition of the new mother is not good, efforts must be made to put everything in normal order already at an early stage.

For the fetus's best, it is very important to start a healthy lifestyle in good time before pregnancy. No smoking should occur and only moderate alcohol con-sumption can be a good advice. Regular exercise and avoidance of stress factors are important. Pregnancy should preferably be checked regularly. Eating the right food is of paramount importance for mother and fetus.

This will be of good help and useful to the expectant mother in order to maintain good health as the unborn child will receive all the nutrients it needs for a healthy development.

It is well known that folic acid should be used 3-4 weeks before, during and after conception to avoid the risk of developing spina bifida.

Spina bifida (a certain form of heredity exists) is a congenital malformation of the vertebrae and their

tagging. This disease occurs in three different forms, hidden Spina bifida occulta (the most common and mildest form), Meningocele and Myelomeningocele, which is the most severe type (spinal cord rock). Folic acid, or vitamin B9 is of good help to build healthy cells.
The body's need for folic acid increases during periods of rapid growth such as pregnancy fetal development.

Research shows that all pregnant women should eat a multivitamin with folic acid, which can reduce the risk of spina bifida by about 70%.
Since spina bifida may develop at the beginning of a pregnancy, often the woman may even not be aware of her condition, it is important to eat folic acid every day. Attending folic acid before and during the early stages of pregnancy, reduces the risk of not only spina bifida but also of other neural defects. Women who wish to become pregnant should eat 0,4 mg of folic acid every day.
A woman having increased risk of spina bifida (a person with a child's pregnancy shawl) should eat 4,0 mg, one to two months before the beginning of pregnancy.

Chlorella which is a good source of folic acid, also provides mother and fetus with other beneficial nutrients that are important for healthy pregnancy including calcium, zinc, selenium and iron as well as with the vitamins A, B, C, D and E which will reduce the risk of anaemia for the pregnant mother.
It is recommended to eat at least 3-6 g of chlorella every day for 1 to 3 months before pregnancy and then continue with the same dose during pregnancy.
3 g chlorella contains about 4,5 mg folic acid.

Chlorella as support for weight control and weight loss.
Obesity is one of the most common health problems affecting a lot of people.
Fortunately, you can take care of it by reducing weight and avoid development of diabetes. If the body's functions are in balance and as digestion and elimination work properly, the body takes on its ideal weight.
In addition, a normalized balance between hunger and nutritional needs of the body occurs. Unfortunately, this natural function is most often interfered with consumed refined food, which today represents a majority of the food in the Western world.
Nutritionally empty calories in sugar, fats, wheat and refined feed, do not provide us with nutrition we need for good health. We eat too little of vegetables and fruit, which would be useful to us. We will be deficient of nutrients and thus we will keep our body in imbalance. For many people, this nutritional deficiency results in unnecessary need for more food that can lead to overweight.
A number of negative effects occur when you eat too much of bad food. It may apply too much of sugar, bad fat and other unhealthy ingredients. Such dieting, for example, refined food and fast food, tends to cause poor combustion, constipation and increased toxic material in the intestinal tract.
In turn, this process prevents proper uptake of vitamins and other vital elements in the diet, which may lead to greater requests for more.
A difficult controlled circuit is created which is easily recognized by those trying to lose weight. What makes it harder is that the secretion of growth hormone decreases in the absence of exercise.

Chlorella is not a "dietary food" that tries to prevent increased appetite. On the other hand, it works to restore balance in the body, so that a correct and permanent improvement as a whole, can be done in terms of good health and weight.

In addition, chlorella may have the importance of participating in a nutritional and effective complement to built a well-balanced weight loss program.

Once, when the intestinal system has been cleaned and can work properly and when the excess material that causes constipation and imbalance has been eliminated, the intestine can again work normally, after which progress can be made to achieve a permanent weight loss.

The doctors Saito and Okano found that Chlorella really stimulated the peristalsis of the intestines and thus contributed to a quick, healthy combustion.

Dr. Bernard Jensen reported and showed that the chlorophyll in chlorella gives this effect.

Chlorophyll in chlorella nourishes the common bacteria of the stomach and it is also known that chlorophyll neutralizes stomach acids. There is no doubt that Chlorella is an effective aid stimulating the peristalsis of the intestinal tract in a well-established weight loss program.

Poor or too slow digestion is often one of the contributing causes of unwanted weight gain and fatness. There are a lot of dieting cures and more or less dubious weight loss programs on the market.

One may however, first think about achieving a good balance in the intestinal tract by means of detoxification processes and consuming healthy and non-acidic diets.

When the intestinal system works normally and has a good bacterial balance, the body can effectively get rid of excessive material that can otherwise contribute to obesity.

Chlorella's beneficial effect on the intestinal peristalsis will immediately help the purification activity that is so important.

Not least essential is that chlorella provides us with a variety of easily absorbable, nutritionally complete substances that are needed in the body and which contribute to a reduced demand for more food.

Dr. Yoshio Yamagashi, head of the *Clinic Hospital of Tokyo, conducted a study in 1961 that involved children who could not digest milk or milk replacement products. Several of the subjects had also allergic reactions. When replacing the milk powder with chlorella, one experienced normal and trouble-free digestion, which shows that chlorella is assimilated safely and easily to people with the most sensitive intestinal systems.*

How to use chlorella by weight loss.

Chlorella can efficiently be used together with any well balanced weight loss program on the market.

Thanks to the ability of chlorella to clean the intestines and stimulate the peristalsis, it can often be enough to contribute to weight loss without having to strictly follow any programs.

Because Chlorella is good food, it does not dampen the appetite.

Instead, Chlorella satisfies the appetite while providing us with energy and a sense of well-being.

Many people in the world who use chlorella pyre-noidosa notice that they are getting reduced desires to eat snacks and sweets and that they simply do not long for it.

There are hundreds of so-called slimming diets and almost as many theories as to lose weight. The experience of most people trying to lose weight is that it is boring and difficult to maintain.

As soon as you finish the diet you begin with old eating habits and a lifestyle that caused the over-weight, thus gaining unwanted weight.

A long-term and necessary weight control involves establishing a lifestyle that includes healthy eating habits, better sleep, positive thinking, and enough of exercise.

In order to achieve the goal of a more effective and sustainable weight reduction and thus improved health, it may be a good idea to eat smaller portions and exercise more than the body previously is used to.

A proper daily diet can contain good, unrefined foods such as whole grain, salads, fresh fruit and vegetable juice or fruit juice.

It means at the same time that you should eat less or preferably to avoid refined sugar, cakes, buns and "heavy" food as beef and pork. There is a reason for desire for junk food to be decreased significantly after a period of time if you regularly enjoy meals with more clean foods. A diet rich in natural food is found to restore the natural balance of the body and help the body to last a long term and avoid weight problems. Chlorella works well with other clean food and helps the body by accelerating the balancing process.

CHLORELLA AND DIFFERENT PROBLEMS.

Allergies

Chlorella's ability to detoxify the body and strengthen the immune system may be helpful against allergies. An allergic reaction occurs when the immune system identifies a potentially harmful substance as an enemy and begins to attack it.

The allergy case can be a hereditary condition, lack of substances that protect the cells and/or an exposure to heavy metals and also depending on too much stress.

Allergy attacks can, for example, be caused by a variety of substances as well by foreign substances such as dust, pollen, fabrics, cosmetics, some foodstuffs, animal fur, mold, chemicals and bacteria.

Allergies usually develop after repeated exposure to substances which, to some extent, initiate a change in body chemistry that causes the production of immunoglobulin E (IgE).

IgE is a group of antibodies that only deal with allergies. IgE bombards the allergen with chemicals that cause symptoms like inflammation, swelling, itching and pain. According to reports, long-term use of chlorella pyrenoidosa has been able to assist against getting hay fever (allergic rhinitis), eczema (atopic dermatitis) and asthma. Another contributing factor may be the immune regulatory activity of the interferon which is increased by the intake of chlorella.

Another reason for allergy prevention can be the increasing number and functions of the body's macrophages. By activating these cells, proteins that cause allergies can be removed faster from the body.

Intestinal purification, enhancement of detoxification mechanism of the liver and the rich content of vitamin A and beta carotene can together contribute to chlorella's anti allergic activity.

Lactose intolerance.
New studies with mice have shown that chlorella extract reduces the production of immunoglobulin (IgE), in the case of milk drinking. It was shown that chlorella extract may be useful in trying to prevent allergic diseases with similar pathology.

In 1997, Japanese researchers conducted a study on children with atopic dermatitis (AD). This skin disease as well as bronchial asthma in children, has increased development in Japan. More than 60% of the children who were assigned were given fifteen to twenty chlorella tablets (3-5 grams daily) during 6 months that clearly showed relieved symptoms of eczema and asthma. It was also found that these children could tolerate milk and eggs significantly better than earlier.

Alzheimer's
Use of aluminum in deodorants and pans has been associated with increased risk of Alzheimer's disease. Regular use of chlorella can help cleanse the body from such heavy metals. Higher oxygen supply to the brain helps the preparedness and mental focus of Alzheimer's patients and for those who suffer from dementia. Studies with chlorella have been conducted in connection with Alzheimer's and dementia. One study showed that among 50 people with Alzheimer's, by the age of 70-90 years who took 6 grams of chlorella pyrenoidosa daily for 6 months, 68% had either stabilized or improved their cognitive functions.

Anemia

Chlorella's richness in chlorophyll stimulates the production of red blood cells and is effective against anemia.
Chlorella has the highest concentration of Vitamin B12, which is a "blood builder", and because of this chlorella is a nutritious food also for vegetarians as there are very few of other non-animal sources of vitamin B12.
Chlorella's fibers and chlorophyll also stimulate the healthy production of the good bacteria in the intestine which produces B12.

Arthritis

Besides its high mineral content, Chlorella is also an alkaline food and can thus help and balance the body pH.
Often our pH level is too acidified as a result of consumption of too much of processed food and carbonated soft drinks. Arthritis is one of the many cases which is associated with an acidified body constitution.

Chlorella's outer cell wall contains glucosamine, which is important for cartilage, tendons, ligaments and other connective tissue.

Autism

Autism is a developmental disorder in children which affects the brain's functions, meaning that the child closes within himself and becomes difficult to reach by the outside world. You do not know the cause of this disease, but heavy metals can be one of more contributing factors. Children with autism are talking later than other children, and as they speak, their communication opportunities are very limited.

They often avoid looking at other people and thus do not learn to read other peoples facial expressions and body languages.

These children can not play creatively but are often self-destructive and start rocking, clapping hands and butting.

Antibodies that are found in autistic children are showing that, in certain cases of autism, it can be caused by a misdirected immune system initiated by a virus.

Researchers at Michigans' College found that autistic children having experiencied attacks by viruses some-times earlier, showed to have higher levels of anti-bodies to brain proteins and suggested an autoimmune reaction.

One has not found any single reason of autism and researchers thought that inheritance factors and environmental factors like viruses and chemicals, could both be of present reasons of the disease.

The type of brain abnormalities that is found in persons with autism, has showed that the disturbance starts when something is disturbing the normal de-velopment of the brain.

One possibility might be that an early exposure of a virus will bring the body to a immunity reaction that in some way is going wrong.

Together with producing antibodies against the virus, the body is producing antibodies against itself, which can result in injuries on tissues and organs.

This autoimmunity reaction is the same as what hap-pens with autoimmune diseases like systemic lupus (SLF) that is a rheumatic disease.

Within scientific circles one states today that autistic children should be avoiding to drink pasteurized milk.

Treatments for autistic symptoms should be to give children food which can be easily assimilated, food that does not cause constipation, food which give them back, the bacteria that help the body to master these inflammatory conditions.

The most important is to try to regain the correct balance with nitrogen and ammonia. The treatments can start by giving the child a healthy diet, rich on proteins like egg, meat, milk (not pasteurized) and cheese and essential fatty acids. Kefir is to prefer to other milk products.

It is a good idea giving the child a daily dose of Chlorella pyrenoidosa as of its possibilities to clean the liver from ammonia, dispatch mercury from the body as well as to be able to clean the intestinal system from poisonous substances.

Chlorella will also assist by increasing the combustion and normalize the intestinal functions moreover that is very important also for the autistic child.

Blood pressures.

Dr. Randall Merchant (Virginia Commonwealth University, USA) is one of the most outstanding experts in chlorella pyrenoidosa.

At a 1998 study, he let patients who wanted to maintain healthy blood pressure take placebo tablets for a month - then chlorella pyrenoidosa for two months.

Results: More than 50% of patients showed similar or better blood pressure values when they took chlorella.

(*Merchant et Al. " Fibromyalgia pilot study of dietary chlorella supplementation," 1998.)*

Cholesterol
In a pilot study where patients ate 9 grams of chlorella each day for one year, they found that they could maintain total serum cholesterol and the harmful LDL at healthy levels without having to change the diet.
("Effects of long-term administration of Chlorella tablets on hyperlipidemia" Jrnl of Japanese Soc. Of Nutr. and Food Science, 1990: 43(3). pp. 167-173)

Digestion
Problems with intestines and stomachs today are a very common problem. Millions of people suffer from stomach pains, loss of appetite, fatigue and lack of body fluids and nutrition.
By a study made the year 1998, patients with different gastrointestinal disorders had chlorella every day for tho months.
90% of the patients received significantly improved intestinal health.
(Merchant, et Al, "Nutritional supplementation with chlorella pyrenoidosa for patients with ulcerative colitis". A pilot study, 1998).

Heart and Circulation
It is very important to maintain strong and healthy blood vessels and it is also the key to a healthy heart and proper circulation.
Chlorella was given to people with problems and after two months, one could discover smoother and more elastic blood vessels in them.

(Chlorella Natural Medicinal Algae by Dr. David Steenblock, page 32 references:

Effects of Chlorella on human pulse wave velocity"
1985, conducted by Kanazawa Medical University, Dep.
of Serology).

Osteoporosis
One of the most prominent problems in women after
menopause is osteoporosis. Osteoporosis also occurs
in men. Women have now learned that they are best
protected from osteoporosis due to intake of extra
calcium and estrogen.
This statement indicates desinformatie in modern
times.
    In our body, bones are living tissues with a rich
network of blood vessels and nerves.
Bones are constantly broken and replaced by special
blood vessels.
Every seventh year, our entire skeleton is replaced.
Bones have a structure that contains calcium and our
legs generally do not suffer from calcium deficiency.
Calcium deficiency results in hypocalcemia (low level
of calcium in the blood).
Serious lack of calcium occurs most in the third world,
were humans have a nutritional deficiency. Body needs
both calcium and magnesium.
Calcium supplements do not increase bone density
before menopause and does not prevent osteoporosis
after menopause. In Scandinavia, England, Australia
and the United States, the most osteoporosis occurs.
In these countries, most milk is consumed by all
countries on Earth.
It is pasteurized milk, cheese and butter that leak our
bone on calcium because these enzyme-free, artificial
and modern nutrients are difficult to metabolize.

Another reason why we lose calcium in the bones and teeth is the consumption of too much acidic food like soft drinks, red meat and white sugar.
All this contributes to acidification in the blood. It is dangerous if the blood is entirely acidified, which can lead to death.
The body's own protection response means that it must neutralize any acid, keeping the pH of the blood between 7,3 to 7,45% which requires calcium.
When insufficient, the body steels calcium from the legs and teeth. This is why Dr. Robert Heaney says, "eating proteinic foods is like letting an acid rain fall on our bones".
It is the wrong protein diet that is the primary cause of osteoporosis.
Factors that can prevent or block the absorption of calcium, include oxalic acid in the diet (spinach, rhubarb, cranberry, lack of vitamin D (sunshine vitamin) overconsumption of protein, salt coffee and alcohol. Likewise, it applies also to soft drinks containing a lot of phosphorus.
Many women with osteoporosis are or have been smokers.

The way to protect yourself from osteoporosis is considered by many researchers, to be eating food that does not acidify the body.
Chlorella pyrenoidosa helps the body to achieve a better balance overall. Chlorella's magnesium, vitamin D and calcium content are effectively absorbed by the body and not least importantly chlorella contributes to normalizing of the pH value.

Chlorella and Cancer.

Treatment with chlorella in connection with various cancers has been tested on both human and animals throughout the years.
Chlorella has shown very good properties for preventive and underlying treatments in these trials. It significantly increases the number of macro-phages and produces an anti-tumor effect and prolongs the lives of human and animals.

It has been shown in recent studies, that another form of white blood cell, the polymorphonuclear leucocyte, is activated by Chlorella extract in a nonspecific way to fight cancer cells.

A recent study indicated that Chlorella derivatives (autoclaves cells and the heat-extracted ones) enhance macrophage activity and cytotoxic activity of lymphocytes (T-cells). The suggestion was made that the anti-tumor action of chlorella was due to a synergistic effect of macrophages and cytotoxic lymphocytes.

Yamaguchi, N., S. Shimizu. T. Murayama, T. Saito, R.F. Wang and Y.C. Tong: Immunomodulation by single cellular algae (Chlorella pyrenoidosa) and anti-tumor activities for tumor bearing mice.
Presented at the Third International Congress of Developmental and Comparative Immunology, Reims, France, July 7-13, 1985

In order to understand chlorella's contributory properties in the fight against cancer, coupling should be directed to the immune system.
Cancer develops with all of us.

As these cancer cells develop, our immune system can destroy them in an efficient and natural way before cancer symptoms develop.

As cancer symptoms appear, it is a clear indication of the immune system's sudden inability to fight cancer cells.

In this way, it can be expressed that the immune system's incapability is directly linked to the development of cancer cells.

Strengthening the immune system should therefore, be one of the most important measures in the fight against cancer development.

Chlorella contains a large number of components that stimulate the immune system that is our build-In defense mechanism. The body has been created with the possibilities to search and destroy abnormal cells that could be highly carcinogenic.

The risk of cancer increases if this ability of our white blood cells (macrophages and T-cells) is weakened due to lack of nutritional support or over-load of excessive levels of free radicals, or other waste.

Animated studies demonstrate that substances in chlorella shows anticancer immunity due to activating of T-cells in the lymphatic system and increasing the availability on these cells into the tumor region. (Tanaka , Noda, Justo).

Daily, chlorella was given in the form of dried powder to tumor-loaded mice. The tumor growth was signi-ficantly reduced in an antigen specific manner me-diated by cytostatic T-cells (Tanaka).

Japanese researchers found that a glycoprotein in chlorella, is a biological defense modifier that shows protection against tumor growth. (Hasegawa).

Cancer refers to more than 100 diseases that attack almost all areas of the body. In a healthy person, cells divide, grow and replace themselves in a methodical way.

As the genes that regulate this cell division fall, cells begin to multiply and spread without control.

Cancer is thus a state where the cells deviate from the normal control of regulated growth and reproduction. These injured cells start multiplying faster than normal and form nodules or tumors.

These may be benign or malignant. Favorable or benign tumors may possibly stop in growth. Malignant tumors, on the other hand, penetrate healthy cells, interfere with bodily functions, exhaust the body's nutrients and spread into the body (metastases). It is the secretion of the dead cellular tissue from the growing cancerous mass, that poison the body's immune system which makes it unable to repel. These cancer cells can spread or form metastases from their place of origin or from other parts of the body via the bloodstream or lymphatic system.

By accelerating the removal of these substances from the body, the immune system becomes more effective in combating the cancer. Causes (or theories about the same) to develop cancer vary and may be completely different for each individual.

Genetic, emotional, environmental and lifestyle factors, all play a roll in different degrees. It is claimed that the genetic impact is 5 to 10%.

What is considered to cause development of cancer?

The majority of cancer cases are considered to be genetic and related to lifestyle factors. However, the real causes of many types of cancer are still unknown. The traditional treatment methods include surgery, chemotherapy and radiotherapy.

Nobel price winner Sir MacFarlane Burnet found that in a normal body, hundreds of cancer cells were formed every day. He considered that it is a normal pheno-menon in the oxidation process and the cellular function. Cancer cells are routinely destroyed by the body's own immune system.

Problems therefore often arise when the immune system is weakened and unable to perform its task.

The majority of cancer cases are not symptomatic. In fact, most are discovered during autopsy. One can say that our current laboratory tests are not sensitive enough to always detect cancer cells. Likewise, it should be emphasized that most cancer cells can not cause any symptoms. In fact, 30 to 40% more cases of thyroid gland-, pancreatic-, and prostate cancer are detected in autopsy than is detected by the physician.

According to a study published in Lancet (British Medical Journal) on February 13, 1993, an early survey is good, but the aggressive nature of traditional medical approach often leads to unnecessary treatment.

In 1992, a study was published in the Journal of the American Medical Association, where 223 patients found that failure to treat prostate cancer could often be better than chemotherapy, radiation, or surgery.

Numerous people develop and die more than ever before and nothing seems to stop developing. Not only does it help through early detection, either to surveys, radiation, surgery or chemotherapy.

The goal of chemotherapy is to gradually reduce the number of cancer cells to the extent that the body's immune response can control continued tumor growth. Sometimes toxic and deadly chemical poisons are used.
Cancer cells are stimulated and struggle to survive in every way by increasing their growth.
Cancer treatment that inhibits the immune system can cause a serious and sometimes life-threatening side effect called leukopenia.

Leukopenia involves an abnormal fall of anti-infectious, circulating white blood cells. Leukopenia not only increases the risk of infection but also delay treatment. The schematic intervals between dosage of chemotherapy are designed to maximize the effect of cancer cells while allowing normal cells to recover. Cancer treatment with chemotherapy seems to "buy time" and often people who have received treatment, experience a temporary relief. In the end, the tumor can return and do it with renewed power.

The body's immune system is designed to fight cancer cells as their growth jeopardizes our organ functions. Our immune system can keep many pro-blems in check as long as it is not compromised by powerful procedures.
Maintaining a strong immune system during the aging process is the key to anti aging, because most cancers are detected after 40 years of age. **Chemotherapy and radiation suppress the immune system just at the time when you most need it.**

Cancer is often a symptom of weakened immune system.

Therefore, it is important to strengthen the immune system and maintain it with the aid of a beneficial lifestyle. It is the best way to search to prevent or delay cancer formation.

Bad eating habits, excessive consumption of carbo-hydrates and trans-fats, lack of exercise, smoking, cancerous environmental hazards, too much of alco-hol, family history, stress and environmental poisoning are the leading reasons.

The biggest contributing causes of cancer are con-sidered to be smoking too much, too much of sun ex-posure too much of stress and a bad diet.

According to Harvard University School of Public Health, the lifestyle is the root cause of 65% of most cancer diseases. Many experts believe that most of these factors lead to an increase in the body's oxidation levels and therefore antioxidants are of great importance with their inhibitors in the fight against cancer diseases.

Stress, although not directly involved to cancer, weakens definitely the immune system, thus increas-ing the risk of cancer. Fortunately, one can control most contributing factors.

If you already have got cancer, you should give the body a chance to better cope with the development of the disease. Maybe you have a chance of getting well.

Many inhibitory factors have been identified by science such as multivitamins, herbs, some foods and, not least, a totally change of lifestyles. In general, traditional treatments often include natural substances extracted from plants, fungi and microorganisms such as algae.

These substances are improving the capacity of the body's own immune system in the way that it remains strong while using traditional treatment methods.

This increases in patients without adversely affecting the effects of the conventional cancer therapy.

Chlorella extracts are well-known in the Japanese scientific world as an immune stimulatory substance.

A number of scientific studies have been able to prove that chlorella represents a healthy benefit for many individuals with impaired immune system caused by disease or chemotherapy. These studies indicate that chlorella accelerates recovery of the immune system, thus increasing resistance to viral infections and enhancing the ability to kill bacteria.

Further, it was discovered that pretreating with chlorella extract could significantly enhance resistance to infection, in part by raised levels of blood cells. Neutrophils are white blood cells that can attract and kill bacteria. Patients who avoid cancer treatment have an increased risk of serious infection because of a too low neutrophil value.

Mice treated with the chemo-therapy drug Cyclophamide received an accelerating recovery of neutrophils when taking chlorella extract.

The white blood cell count was one and a half to two times higher in comparison with the control group.

Growth and differentiation of white blood cells depend on particular proteins produced by the body and are called colony stimulating factors (CSF). Chemical messengers called cytokines mobilize immune cells.

Chlorella can increase growth and activity in white blood cells by stimulating the secretion of CSF and different cytokines.

(Effect of hot water extract of Chlorella on cytokines expression patterns in mice with murine acquired immuno-deficiency syndrome after infection with Listeria Mono-cyhtogenes, Immuno-pharmacology, 1997; 35:pp 273-282)

Fatty diet
There is very strong evidence of correlation between a high trans-fat diet and a variety of types of cancer, especially in the breast-, colon and prostate gland. Recent studies have shown increased risk of intestinal cancer through trans fats, especially from hydrolyzed vegetarian oils.

Alcohol consumption.
Researchers at Harvard School of Public Health analyzed a study involving 320000 women.
It was found that women who drank two to five alcoholic drinks a day were at greater risk of developing breast cancer than those who were absent from alcoholic drinks.
It was also found that even a lesser consumption of alcohol, perhaps one drink, increased the risk of cancer by about 9%.

Physical inactivity.
In a study of 25624 women, researchers found that the lowest risk of cancer occurred in light weight persons who exercised at least four hours a week.
Obesity
As a common side effect of physical inactivity and excessive intake of carbohydrates, constitutes in itself a risk factor for certain types of cancer.

Researchers found a connection between overweight women before menopause and mortality of breast cancer. Today, it is also considered that type 2 diabetes is a direct consequence of over-weight obesity.

Undernourishment

40 percent or more of cancer patients die of malnutrition. Percussion of cancer is subject to threefold threats.
1. Having bad appetite and not eating enough
2. The body uses more nutrition than ever before.
3. Their nutritional needs have increased dramatically.

The following are just a part of known cancer suppressing nutrients.

Folic acid.

Recent studies show that folic acid, a B-vitamin, can reduce the risk of breast cancer in women who drink alcoholic beverages.
However, it should be taken into consideration that for people who drink too much, folic acid has not directly a positive impact, but instead lose its beneficial effect. Recommended intake of folic acid is 400 micrograms per day. Chlorella contains folic acid.

Coenzyme Q10,

Q10 is located next to all living cells, especially in mitochondria (energy factors). Q10 is considered to provide some protection against breast cancer.

C-vitamin

C-vitamin may be thought to protect against side effects from certain anticancer drugs. A daily intake of 250 mg is recommended. Chlorella contains C-vitamin.

Omega-3 As an essential fatty acid, omega-3 can protect against skin cancer tumors. In order to have a good health effect, one is recommended 1% to 2.5% of daily calorie intake. Chlorella contains omega-3.

Carotenoids.
Carotenoids are transformed into vitamin A by the body's needs. They contain lutein, zeaxanthin, beta-cryptoxanthin, lycopene, alpha-carotene and beta-carotene. A lack of carotenoids can increase risk of breast cancer. Chlorella is a carotenoid.

Vitamin E
Vitamin E is beneficial in the treatment of skin cancer. It has shown that the natural form of alpha toco-pherols has a better absorption capacity than synthe-tically produced vitamin E. Chlorella contains vitamin E in natural form.

There are more than 100 types of cancer that vary in symptoms and aggressiveness.
One can divide most cancer into four categories:
Carcinoma: cancer that affects the skin, mucous membranes, glands and internal organs.
Leukemia: blood vessel cancer
Sarcoma: muscle cancer, connective tissue and bone.
Lymphoma: Cancer of the lymphatic system.

Some type of cancer takes about 20 years to develop. The conclusion is that slowly an unnoticed and gradual concomitant degenerative change of tissue occurs.
We get it by destroying the chemical balance in the body so that cell repair can't happen because we do not supply the body with cellular materials.

At the end of the 1980s, cancer cells were found to invade normal tissues through the use of specific enzymes, (endoglycosidase, cathepsin B, plaminogen activator and the major type IV collagen).
This is a fundamental process that allows cancer cells to spread through the body and possibly lead to the death of the patient.

Usually, it is not the original cancer that kills a human but the "small seeds" of cancer that spread and invades other tissues to grow.
Chlorophyll has been shown to have antiproteolytic activities (preventing muscle tissue burning).
Chlorella is the largest source of chlorophyll which can play an important role in attempting to treat cancer spread (metastasis) by seeking to prevent these cancer cells' protein metabolism enzymes.

Chlorella increases the number of macrophages in mice with tumor formation due to an anti-tumor effect that is an extension of animal life.
Other recent studies have shown that another form of blood cell (polymorphonuclear leukocytes) is activated by the intake of chlorella extract (CGF) to inevitably counteract cancer cells.
Another recent study showed that chlorella derivatives, especially (autoclaved cells from the hot water extract), enhances the lymphocytes (possibly T-cells) macrophage activity and cytotoxic activity.
The thought arose that chlorella's anti-tumor activity was due to synergistic effects in macrophages and cytotoxic lymphocytes.
Vermeil and Morin were the first to prove this relationship and that the material in chlorella's cell wall could have a clear influence on cancer.

They demonstrated that injections with chlorella in the abdomen protected CH3 mice to 82% against sarcoma BP8 tran-splantation.
The group's continued work showed that anti-tumor effect could inevitably be due to the stimulus of the macrophages.

An acidic polysaccharide made from Chlorella's cell wall has been shown to stimulate the production of interferon both in test tubes and experimental mice.
The induced interferon is capable of protecting the mice from infections by vaccines and influenza viruses, and has also demonstrated anti-tumor activity against Ehrlich disease.
In addition, it has been discovered that the consti-tuents of the polysaccharides in Chlorella's cell wall are effective against cancer, at least in part, due to its stimulus to interferon production.

CGF stimulates the production of interferon which is considered to decrease the growth of cancer cells.
Interferon is a natural secretion in the body and is considered to be a fusion stimulator for the functions of macrophages. Injections of interferon enhance the macrophages' function and metabolism. Mechanism in Chlorella Immune stimulants may seem similar to the activity of interleukin I and Il on lymphocytes by activating the cells to become more active.
Chlorella stimulates the activity of T-cells and macrophages by raising the level of interferon, thereby promoting the immune system's ability to counteract foreign invaders, whether they are bacteria, viruses, chemicals or promotional pro-teins.

Additionally, it appears that chlorella's cell wall has the ability to fight cancerous cells by interferon production induced by complex polysaccharides.

Chlorella's unique cell wall is one of the important factors that distinguish chlorella from other "green" food.

Chlorella increases the production of T-cells and B-cells.

B-cells and T-cells in the body are active against viruses and cancer. The macrophages are large cells surrounding and destroying foreign substances in the body. They are active against cancer, foreign proteins and chemicals.

Chlorella can stimulate macrophages and T-cells in the immune system, which causes anti-effect because they can maintain their activity, which otherwise usually weakens in the body as the cancer tumor begins to grow.

(According to a combined report from the Kanazawa Medical Unit, Taipei Medical University at the Third International Congress in Reims, France, 1985).

Mice injected with cancer cells showed higher resistance to these when they had been administrated with chlorella. Other trials showed that chlorella's growth factor (CGF) enhances the defense of abdominal cancer by increasing the number of immune cells in the abdominal cavity.

Chlorella extract injected into mice with Sarcoma 180 (cancer cells) prolonged the life of the animals significantly. (Experiments at Kitazato Institute).

Chlorella supports cell reproduction, reduces cholesterol and increases hemoglobin levels.

Through its broad nutrition and detoxification profile, it facilitates repair of body organs and damaged tissues. Chlorella's stimulatory effect on the liver and other detoxifying organisms had not been studied in relation to metastatic cancer, but the ability to work to purify the blood from cancer cell spills, could be real because algae stimulates the removal of foreign substances and other bad and unhealthy subjects from the blood.

In the treatment of cancer patients, the number of some lymphocytes and their relationship to each other is of importance (cell proportion helper/killer). Cancer patients have often lowered level of helper cells and elevated levels of killer cells.

High doses of chlorella have been shown to reverse this ratio in some patients, a decrease of killer cells and an increase of helper cells. This has been demonstrated in patients with Hodgkin's disease already after 6 weeks of chlorella treatment.

A number of scientific reports have shown that chlorella, with the exception of chlorophyll derivative (photo-dynamic therapy), do not have direct activity against any cancer or tumor.

What has instead been shown is that chlorella, either given orally or through injections, develops significantly anticancer activity by stimulating the carrier's own immune system.

This simply means that chlorella stimulates and strengthens the body's own immune system so that it can combat cancer more effectively.

Anticancer activity appears to be present in both chlorella's cell wall (which are composed of acidic polysaccharides) and within the cells as its water soluble extract has also been shown to have anti-cancer activity.

1990 a publication (Pbytotherapy Research 1990; 4: 220 231) published clinical trials with chlorella at the Medical Collage of Virginia.

Dr. Randall Merchant with colleagues gave chlorella to patients with different types of lethal brain-tumors (malign glioma).

These patients had advanced and conventionally not curable brain-tumors, possibly with fatal outcome within a maximum of one year.

After 2 years of study of patients taking chlorella in both tablets and CGF in big doses, 7 patients out of 20 survived. These 7 patients showed no more signs of their cancer. During the 2 years, patients received daily 20 grams of chlorella tablets and 150 ml of chlorella growth factor (CGF). The high dose did not produce any side effects or other toxic reactions. Blood tests and MRI/CT scanners were used for each patient. During the test period, the patients had over all, less infections or other flulike illnesses than expected in their respiratory systems.

The majority of patients explained that chlorella helped them maintain power and strength. The red blood vessel value was normal for 18 of the 20 patients. (Data published 1990. Plytotherapy Research Vol. 4 No. 6 pp. 220-231).

Chlorella helps the body to quickly rebuild the white blood cells to counteract fatigue during chemotherapy.
How much chlorella can a cancerous person eat?

It is not uncommon for a cancerous person to eat as much as 20-30 grams per day. A person with skeletal cancer showed very good results after 6 months with a 20 grams of chlorella intake per day.

The most positive results showed when 60 to 90 ml of CGF were taken at the same time with about 30 grams of chlorella in tablet or powder form.
In all cases, nutritionally oriented medical should be consulted.

Chlorella, Beta carotene and cancer cells. Chlorella contains 180 mg beta carotene per 100 grams.

Chlorella contains 180 mg beta carotene per 100 grams.
The fact that chlorella can support the body to fight cancer has been shown in scientific studies of vitamin-A and beta carotene's cancer-inhibiting prospects.
There are thousands of documents showing vitamin-A and beta carotene's effects on the immune system, both in the prevention and direct treatment of cancer.

Simply explained, vitamin-A affect the immunity by:

1 Maintaining the mechanical integrity of tissues and mucous membranes such as mouth coating, esophagus, intestines and skin.

2 Acting as an unspecified healthy tonic.

3 Being stimulating to the phagocytes of the body to attack foreign intruders and cancer cells.

People who develop cancer have shown, that they often have lower levels of A-vitamin in the blood. People who regularly eat a lot of vegetables and fruits, are less likely to get cancer due to the high content of A-vitamin in the diet. As high doses of A-vitamin is combined with radiation therapy in cancer treatment, the dose of radiation can be reduced by 50% which means that the patient can tolerate radiation doses with minor side effects.

The Robert Janker clinic in Bonn, Germany was pioneering when it comes to using high doses of A-vitamin in cancer treatment.
In 1971, the group published the results of 37 cases of cancer in the vulva, the patients being treated with high doses of A-vitamin and radiation.
Radiation rates were reduced to 1/3 compared with those treated solely with radiotherapy.
Similar results were found in the treatment of throat cancer. At the 14th International Cancer congress in Budapest in 1986, Dr. Wolfgang Scheef informed at the Janker Clinic about his results 20-year results of the use of high doses of emulsified A-vitamin on patients.
He reported an almost 100% cure of mild skin cancer as well as clearly demonstrated good results in treating a number of other cancer types. Beta carotene has the largest A-vitamin and anti-oxidant activity of all known carotenoids. Beta carotene helps to defend the body against free radicals and has been shown to   destroy cancer cells and enhance the production of macrophages as well as interleukin I (T-helper cell stimulator). Beta carotene works syner-gistically with E-vitamin as an antioxidant to combat cancer at an early stage.

Chlorella extract can provide good support in conventional cancer treatment.
The goal of chemotherapeutic treatment is to gradually reduce the number of cancerous cells to the extent that the body's own immune system can take control of cancer growth.

In order to achieve this, chemotherapy is directed against cells that often divide, as is the case with cancerous cells.

Unfortunately, this also affects on what the body is dependent for the fight against cancer, namely of white blood cells.

Cancer treatment that suppresses the immune system can cause a serious and sometimes life-threatening side effect such as leukopenia (too low of white blood cells).

Leukopenia not only increases the risk of infection but may also delay the cancer treatment. The planned intervals between dosages of the chemotherapy, are intended to maximize the effect on the cancer cells while normal healthy cells can be reset.

Delay of treatment may prevent progress toward disease due to abnormally low white blood cells.

Research studies have shown that patients, with impaired immune systems, caused by disease or chemotherapy treatment, can benefit significantly from the intake of Chlorella. In these studies, it has been shown that chlorella can strengthen resistance to viral infections and improve the body's own ability to kill bacteria.

(Protective effect of an acidic glycoprotein obtained from culture of chlorella against myelosuppression by 5-fluorouracil, Cancer Immunology, Immunotherapy, June 1996, 42:pp. 268-741).

Neutrophils are white blood cells that have the ability to ingest and kill bacteria. Patients who fail cancer treatment have an increased risk of serious infections due to low neutrophil count.

Mice treated with chemotherapy medication, Cyclophospharmide, received accelerating recovery of neutrophils when given chlorella.
When experimental mice were injected with E. coli bacteria, the mice treated with chlorella showed a remarkably increased incidence of white blood cells to the infection area.
(Enhanced resistance to Escherichia coli infection by subcutaneous administration hot water extract of chlorella vulgaris in cyclo-phosphamide-treated mice, Cancer Immunology, Immunotherapy, 1990; 32 pp. 1-7)

Growth and differentiation of white blood cells depends on particular proteins produced by the body and called colony stimulating factor (CSF). Chemical messengers called cytokines mobilize immune cells.
Chlorella can increase growth and activity in white blood cells by stimulating the secretion of CSF and different cytokines.
(Effect of hot water extract of Chlorella on cytokine expression patterns in mice with murine acquired immunodeficiency syndrome after infection with Listeria Monocytogenes, Immunopharmacology 1997; 35: pp, 273-282).

Under a study (1990) at the University of Virginia in USA, individuals with seemingly unbearable cases of brain tumors received a daily intake of chlorella in high doses.
All patients could, despite their severe brain tumor disease, for a long time, retain a significantly higher quality of life by daily eating high doses of chlorella.

The patients had a smaller frequency of infections than in other cancer patients, and after 2 years, 30% of the patients were still alive.

The American medical doctor and researcher, Dr. David Steenblock treated, among others, a patient with lymhoma cancer whose blood image clearly improved after daily intake of 27 grams of Chlorella pyrenoidosa for 6 weeks.

Numerous studies point to tumor-inhibiting and life-saving properties of Chlorella pyrenoidosa. For many years, we have been aware of chlorella's stimulation on the immune system by the ability to attract heavy metals and foreign bodies to the body and expel them through the intestinal tract. At the same time, chlorella supplies the body a variety of essential nutrients that, in conjunction with detoxification processes, strengthen the immune system, enhancing the body's self-healing properties.

Circulation
Chlorella assist us to counteract stress factors (adaptogen). Stress releases hormones like cortisol, which effects circulation and causes many other problems in our body. Chlorella assists us by normalizing the flow of our body. Around 15% of the flow in our body is blood and the lymphatic system carries out further 70%.
The blood is transported in the body through the circulatory system and with the help of the heart pump. Both systems are vital to the body's health condition.

If flow of blood through the body is in any way prevented, its ability to function is impaired to function
and we become susceptible to debilitating effects.
Common symptoms include a feeling of heaviness in
the arms or difficulty reversing the head. These
problems are often caused by a blockade of lymphatic
flow.
The superior nutritional balance in chlorella assists to
facilitate and normalize the flow of essential fluids in
our metabolic pathways. In particular, chlorella dis-
courages some of the problems that occur in adults in
a sedentary lifestyle or malnutrition.
These effects arise from problems with the flow of
body fluids through our metabolic pathways such as
bloodstream or lymph.
It is therefore essential that we have a good flow in
our bloodstream that can help us prevent problems
caused by a deteriorating lifestyle.

Cardiovascular health
Chlorella is the riches natural source of chlorophyll.
Chlorophyll cells have a structure similar to that of hemoglobin.
The only difference is that chlorophyll cells have a
magnesium (Mg) molecule in their core, hemoglobin
has iron (Fe) in its centre.
    Magnesium is essential for heart health and is also
known to be beneficial to high blood pressure and
other body systems.
Chlorella also provides us with omega 3 fatty acid,
which is known to be a good protection against heart
disease.
Research programs have indicated that regular use of
chlorella's protective effect on heart disease, contri-

butes to normalization of high blood pressure and lowers high blood cholesterol levels. (Merchant)

Chlorella and the liver.
There exist many reasons for liver cirrhosis (cells that die and are replaced by connective tissue), also called fat liver.
This condition is also called cirrhosis. Other diseases can also result cirrhosis which causes the blood circulation deteriorate to the liver, the pressure increases in the portal vein and varicose veins can occur in the lower part of the esophagus.

As a consequence of the high pressure, new veins are formed that lead the bloodstream past the liver. Some of these veins can form a spinal cord in the gastrointestinal tract. Varicose can burst and cause bleeding. In addition it could cause jaundice, weather in the abdominal cavity and nervous system, or that gives symptoms that can cause fainting and is called liver dysfunction.
Portal hypertension also causes the blood to accumulate in the spleen which then becomes larger and destroys more platelets than normal.

It is not so common with primary malignant tumors in the liver, whereas tumors from other organs are more common.
Primary tumor is more often located in the gastrointestinal tracts.
One of the most common causes of fatty liver, in addition to alcohol abuse, is nutritional deficiency (especially in the case of amino acids with sulfur content).
Diabetes can cause a type of fat liver and excessive consumption of refined carbohydrates, can cause another one.

Attempts have been made in the Republic of China, Japan and Germany to investigate the effects that chlorella could have on preventing various liver conditions.

The trials showed very promising and positive results. One of the first comparative studies on the effect of algae and other foodstuffs (skimmed milk powder and boiled egg whites) on the liver was performed in the 1950s in Germany at the universities of Bonn and Cologne.

Dr. Hermann Fink gave groups of rats different diets to be able to observe how algae compared to other known nutrients could affect health.

Most rats assigned skimmed milk died of liver cirrhosis while a rat eating egg-white showed signs of cirrhosis. All rats that had eaten algae remained in good health. Dr. Fink stated that further research would be conducted to investigate the therapeutic impact of green algae on the liver.

Chlorella protects the liver.
Several trials have shown that chlorella stimulates the protective effects on the liver and the organ's resistance and risk of degradation due to toxins. Chlorella lowers blood cholesterol and triglycerides whose levels are associated with liver metabolism as well as fat intake. We find that chlorella has a protective and purifying effect on the liver and supports the body's own natural defense.

In 1975, Japanese scientific researchers published an article in the Japanese Journal of Nutrition, which showed that chlorella lowered both blood cholesterol and liver cholesterol. It showed that chlorella has a definitive positive effect on liver functions.

H and E. Herold Fink "The protein value of Unicellular Green Algae and Their Action in Preventing Necrosis". Zeitschrift Phystoll. Chem. 305 (1956).

The German study shows that the liver received the protection from injuries caused by malnutrition.
Like chlorella's remarkable levels or chlorophyll which successfully binds and supports the removal of environmental pollutants, this single-cell alga contains additional properties that work synergistically with chlorophyll, thus facilitating detoxification of the liver and enhancing its functional properties.
　　Especially essential is that Chlorella contains glutathione which is the key component of the face II of the detoxification process of the liver.

Glutathione is in CGF (Chlorella Growth Factor) a combination of nutritious and functional components which are showing a lot of medical properties.
In another hospital, Chlorella and CGF were given to patients with far advanced wound formation which refused to heal with commonly used medication and treatment. New tissues were discovered after a couple of days and all sores had soon healed completely. In its case it turned out that, as the body's own resources were tired and weakened, the addition of Chlorella and CGF had a functional ability to stimulate a faster repair of the tissue.

The stomach ulcers and other hard-to-treat wounds were also mentioned here, but in none of these cases, the results could be attributed to constituting any particular diet or other medical treatment, as it clearly showed that new tissues were first formed when treatment with Chlorella was started.

Many other diseases and conditions have been improved after Chlorella has been given to patients in the above mentioned cases, which is sufficient evidence to show that there is one or more nutrients in Chlorella that contribute to the repair of cells and tissues.

Chlorella Growth Factor (CGF) and glutathione.

CGF is considered to be a concentrate in the chlorella gene's nucleotide and comprised of nucleic acid-associated substances, peptides, proteins, amino acids, vitamins and sugars.

Of particular interest and taking detoxification into account is the presence of peptide glutathione in the chlorella growth factor (CGF).

Matsueda S et al. 1982 Studies on anti tumor active glycoprotein from Chlorella, Yajugaku-Zassh (102:447-51).

Glutathione is a powerful detoxification molecule that plays an important role in phase II in the detoxification process. One fact is, that exposure of environmental pollutants reduces the body's stock of glutathione while nutritional food as chlorella can achieve the opposite by stimulating the body's ability to get rid of toxic chemicals. Additionally, Chlorella pyrenoidosa contains an extensive range of nutritional compounds that work synergistically to support the process of environmental detoxification in the body.

Chlorella and our intestinal system.

Among the body's organs, the intestines are most susceptible to disease but do not always show signs of nuisance.

Unfortunately, it is in the intestines that the basic disease-inducing factors occur. We may be unaware of these factors, as they can be difficult to detect for many years before it leads to sudden onset of symptoms of chronic or degenerative disease.
The intestinal tract of intestines is compromised by chronic mineral deficiency and toxic accumulation, which may not be accompanied by symptoms at an early stage of development.

When chlorella is eaten regularly for a prolonged period, tissue functions are raised to their optimal level of integrity by algae supporting correction of mineral deficiency, prevent accumulation and repairing damaged tissue
We find that the intestines have such few pain sensitive nerves that many different kinds of serious problems can develop there without the usual warning signs such as pain and discomforts and which also signal problems in most other parts of the body.
Extreme gas formation, constipation or diarrhea can cause swelling, cramps, uncomfortable pressure on the stomach and other symptoms but most other intestinal conditions do not reveal symptoms until severe consequences have developed in the body.

Chlorella's cell wall acts to absorb toxins in the intestine and promote normal intestinal movements.
The intestinal walls, especially in the small intestine, have spots of lymphocytes that are likely to be stimulated by the material in chlorella cell wall to strengthen its ability to destroy bacteria.
Chlorella also stimulates the growth of the good bowel bacteria (lactic acid bacteria) and others that produce vitamin B12.

Chlorella's stimulating and detoxifying abilities of the intestinal tract, usually show interesting results. A number of people who start taking chlorella, experience more gases than usual during the first 3 to 7 days.

This condition is believed to be due to the fermentation and neutralizing of the harmful bacteria. After this initial period, the intestines will work better than before and the problem of extra gas formation will decrease completely.

What you notice is that chlorella, containing most of chlorophyll of all plants in the world, contributes to reducing the odor from the stool, which can be explained by a better and more normalized ph in the body and that the process of decay becomes more efficient and also shortened time-wise.

All organs are influenced by the intestines.
The known Dr John Harvey Kellogg described many cases when surgery procedures were considered unnecessary due to the remediation and revitalization of the intestines.

Dr Kellogg considered that 90% of modern civilization's diseases are caused by weak intestinal function.

The relationship between under-activity in the intestine and disease is supported by Sir Arbuthnot Lane from London, who considered that the lower part of the intestine is of such order that it is considered to need to be emptied every six hours, but instead and maybe by habit, we may retain its contents under maybe up to 24 hours or more. The result may be either stomach ulcer and risk of cancer.

Later on, the British surgeon Dr Dennis Burkitt found, after many years of work and medical studies in East Africa, that Africans living in the the countryside, did not have any problems with over-fatness, diabetes, hernia, appendicitis, diverticulosis, ulcerative colitis, polyps or intestinal cancer.

Dr Burkitt attributed much of the merit to this by regularly eating a diet rich in fiber, fresh fruit, vegetables, and grains that keep the intestine clean which makes the food transport faster and more efficient through the intestinal tract.

The problem is to eat a lot of modern junk food, refined foods, fast food and lack of exercise, all together contributing to slow intestinal activity to the extent that toxic chemical reactions, depletion, severe gas formation and absorption of toxins through the intestinal walls, provide good grounds for disease.

Toxic substances are absorbed by blood flow and lymph from which they can settle in the congenital weak organs and tissues of the body.

As this continues over the years, the weakest organs break down first, just as the weakest link in a chain can break.

Due to the fact that the intestine can affect so many other body tissues in this way without displaying symptoms, it can be said, that problems in the heart, liver, lungs, kidneys and many other organs are often treated without recognizing and treating the original source to the problem - a toxic, under-active intestine.

Of all the body's elimination system, the intestine is always the first to become under-active and poisoned, which in turn increases the burden on the other excretory organs like the lymphatic system and liver.

Unless the intestine is clean and active, we can not maintain pure blood and lymph and since blood and lymph are contaminated, all organs, glands and tissues in the body are affected.

Due to the interdependence of organs, a serious problem in one of them may be a contributing cause of problems in other organs.
A toxic bowel can therefore be a disability even for the strongest organ in the body.
   Any remediation process or substance that can help to regularly detoxify the intestine is beneficial to the entire body. Statistics show that we generally use 30% or more of wheat products, 25% to 30% milk products, and 10% to 12% of refined sugar.
In total, it will be about 70% or more of decaying food as it would instead be as low as 6%. More healthy would be to use more fresh fruit, vegetables and whole grains (other than wheat) in the daily diet.

Excessive overdose means disaster for the relationship of proper nutrition and the health of the body.
Wheat, especially refined white flour products, contain gluten which tends to coat and irritate the small intestine, reduce assimilation of nutrition and contribute to a slow and sluggish intestine. A similar excessive use of milk products can also contribute to slow intestinal, constipation and cataract formation while high sugar consumption contributes to worsening of the intestine and increased acidification in the body.
Some people are affected more than others of these states. But in any case and at high consumption of these three products, deficiencies develop because there is not enough nutrition in the diet.

We can not built a healthy body with a diet consisting of 60-70% white floor, milk and sugar.
One of the biggest problems with white floor, milk and sugar is that they do not contain any fibers, the hard-melted vegetarian cellulose that condition and provide with exercise to the intestinal walls, absorbs moisture and reduces the time of transport through the intestine.

The longer time the food waste is used to get through the intestine, the more it leads to fatigue and gas formation. Swelling of intestines, diverticulosis and thickening of the intestinal mucosa are formed.

The intestine becomes a stationary sewage line that contaminates the rest of the body. Exercise can compensate for bad eating habits to a degree, but not enough. We need both good eating habits and regular exercise to make the bowel function and work better. Exercise improves digestion and keeps the intestine more flexible.

The regularity of the intestine is positively affected by regular exercise.

Despite today's modern "work out" facilities that are popular with primarily younger people, middle aged and older people do not get enough exercise, although they belong to the group that needs it in particular.

Exercise does not necessarily have to be linked to expensive tools and training locations. Outdoors quick walks with varying speed and swimming are two of the best kind of exercise programs we can do, according to the expertise. We can not repair a toxic intestine overnight but we can start by giving the bowel a healthy nutrition as a starter.

There are four components of chlorella that accelerate the process of cleansing and detoxification. When used in combination with natural, fiber rich diet and also a daily intake of, for example kefir, chlorella can produce tremendous results for the intestinal system.

The four ingredients are chlorophyll, Chlorella growth factor (CGF), protein and fibers which are working in harmony with the treatment of the intestine.

Chlorophyll is the most effective cleaning agent you can find in nature! When you begin to detoxify the intestine, you simultaneously clean the liver, kidneys and blood flow, strengthen the intestinal flora and relieve irritated tissue along the intestinal wall.

CGF accelerates healing in the intestinal wall, while the chlorella protein is immediately available for repair and recovery of damaged tissue, whereas RNA contained in large amounts in chlorella, accelerates the healing process.

Japanese medical research and personal evidence show that chlorella stimulates peristalsis and activates the intestine to an increased degree of remediation. As the intestines are under-active, not only the blood flow but also the other detoxification channels are overloaded when they replace intestinal missing features.

As this continues over the years, the weakest organs are broken down first just like the first weak link in a chain.

The average capacity of our detoxification organ determines the activity rate of the lymphatic system. When the detoxifying agents are under-active, it is usually too much toxic material that circulates in the body so that the liver gets difficult to be detoxified.

There will also be too much toxic material to carry away for the lymphatic system and thus too much for the natural immune system. The body's defense is therefore reduced!

You can not detoxify the intestinal system overnight, but you can make a healthy start of the process itself. Chlorophyll in chlorella is nature's most effective cleaning and detoxifying substance. Chlorophyll begins the process of detoxifying the intestine, the kidneys, liver and blood flow, nourishing the the intestinal flora and calm irritated tissue along the intestinal walls. When you begin to eat chlorella, it may occasionally occur that you therefore experience an initial reaction such as gas formation or loose stool for 3 to 7 days. This is because the intestinal system begins to be cleaned and detoxified. Such positive reactions indicate the ability of chlorella to restore body balance.

One of the first findings is that chlorella pyrenoidosa stimulates and normalizes an under-active intestinal system.

Dr. Motomichi Kobayashi, head of a hospital in Takamatsu, Japan prescribes chlorella pyrenoidosa for all his patients suffering from constipation.

An American Army Institution in Colorado discovered that when chlorella pyrenoidosa was given to a group of volunteers, the level of waste that was eliminated by the intestines of these individuals increased. In 1957, Dr. Takechi and his research team discovered that chlorella caused faster growth of lactobacilli, one of the bacteria that contributes to better bowel functions.

Chlorella chlorophyll helps to keep the intestine clean while chlorella's strong cellulose membrane (which is not digestible) binds to mercury, cadmium, lead and other heavy metals and expels them from the body.

Chlorella growth factor stimulates repair of tissue damage.

Summary of Chlorella's good properties for the intestine is, that chlorella regenerates regularity and balances in the intestine, normalizes beneficial intestinal flora, helps with detoxification and stimulates repair of damaged tissues.

It is important to note that chlorella pyrenoidosa enhances the body's ability to eliminate toxins through all four detoxification channels. This contributes to to the rebuilding and rejuvenation of the natural defense system as a whole, and in particular, to the immune system.

Chlorella helps to clean blood flow.
A pure blood flow with a large number of red blood cells that can produce oxygen is necessary for a strong natural immune system. Chlorella's cleansing effect on the intestine and other elimination channels as well as its ability to protect the liver, also helps to purify the blood. Pure blood ensures that metabolic waste is removed from the tissues.

The structure of metabolic toxins in the body is likely to be as serious a problem as the accumulation of toxic material from the unhealthy food, contamination and exposure to chemicals in workplaces and other environments.

Chlorella helps to balance blood sugar.

Many studies have shown that chlorella appears to normalize blood glucose levels, both in cases of low blood sugar and high blood sugar levels, and which in the latter case can lead to diabetes. Proper sugar levels are important in order to have normal brain function, cardiac function and energy metabolism all of which are necessary to maintain good health and prevent disease.

The liver and pancreas are involved in the regulation of blood sugar, especially insulin-producing gland cells that lie as islets in the pancreas (insula is Latin for "islets").

It has been found that chlorella supports and balances pancreatic gland functions as well as functions of other organs mentioned above.

Chlorella and colds.

A large-scale experiment with chlorella was performed on nearly one thousand Japanese seaman who were on a trip from Japan to Australia and back for about 95 days.

Two grams of chlorella were distributed daily to 485 randomly selected crew members, while 513 others who did not receive chlorella, served as a comparison group. About 30% fewer cases of cold and flu appeared in the group assigned to chlorella. A substance called "clone A" extracted from chlorella's nuclear material stimulates interferon production and helps protect the cells against viruses.

Chlorella stimulates normalization of blood pressure.

It has been known for many years that chlorella helps to normalize blood pressure mentioned in many documented cases. High blood pressure is known to be one of the main risk factors for heart attack and stroke, which causes more deaths than any other disease in many countries. Laboratory experiments have shown that regular use of chlorella lowers blood pressure and prevents stroke. Cases of low blood pressure are not so extensive, but when chlorella has been used for a few months, blood pressure is more well balanced and normalized.

Chlorella helps in wound healing.
In Japan, chlorella has long been used to try to heal difficult wounds. Japanese doctors found that difficult ulcers were healed faster using chlorella. This also showed that wounds that did not respond to varying conventional medical treatment, were finally healed when patients received chlorella and CGF supplementation. Research trials have shown that a substance in CGF (chlorella growth factor) stimulates faster reproduction, which contributes to more efficient healing.
Many doctors and researchers believe that only nutrition can build new tissues and that it is the secret of proper and effective healing.

Medical experiences with chlorella.
Good results with chlorella have been detected in symptoms of chronic gastritis and gastric ulcer. At Saito Hospital, Fukuoka, Japan, doctors used chlorella in patients with stomach ulcers and gastrointestinal ulcers, which have failed to heal with commonly used medication. Most of above problems and pains also disappeared within 10 days.
Other symptoms disappeared totally after 10 to 21 days. X-rays showed complete healing in most cases.

A miniature camera confirmed that new tissues had enclosed the wounds. (From Yamagishi, Yoshio, "The treatment of Peptic Ulcers by use of chlorella" Nibon iji shimpo, No. 1997 (1962)

Chlorella and Vitamin B12
Vitamin B12 has probably the most complex composition of all vitamins and is also not so easily accessible through the diet.
Chlorella is a good source of vitamin B12 which is accessible to the body and chlorella provides us with more of this vitamin than ox liver.
According to well-known researcher, Dr. Dhyana Bewicke, "3 grams of chlorella gives us about 70% of the daily requirement of vitamin B 12".

Dr. Joel Schwartz, Dr. Diana Suda and Dr. Gerald Shklar at Harvard School of Dental Medicine reported following research findings at the 1986 Academy of Oral Pathologist meeting in Toronto, Canada.

Results showed an effect with beta carotene on carcinogenic cancer in hamsters having been injected with carcinogen 7.12- Dimethylbenzanthracene.
Chlorella extracts were also studied, which proved it to have a greater effect than beta-carotene alone, which prompted the group to wonder whether or not other factors exist in chlorella which could give the algae greater anti-tumor activity than could be expected with only beta carotene content.

Age-related macular degeneration (age changes in the yellow spot).

When you read this text, you are using the part of the retina, called macula. The macula adds clarity and color to the eyesight.

Age-related macular degeneration is the main cause of visual impairment in people over 55 years of age.

Until recently, changes in the yellow spot were accepted as an inevitable aging process.

Research shows however, that the problem in question, can be linked to nutritional deficiencies. By increasing the intake of certain nutrients, you can prevent or stop the cause of vision impairment. In particular, lutein represents a promising nutritional therapy for treating and preventing age changes in the yellow spot. Lutein is a member of a nutrition group called carotenoids. The most famous member is beta carotene which chlorella has a rich content of.

Carotenoids are distributed through the body in various proportions.

Chlorella's anti-inflammatory properties.

Scientific research at the Department of Pathology, Oklahoma State University Center for Health Sciences investigated the incidence of anti-inflammatory properties of chlorella.

The researchers found inhibitory release of histamine from stem cells. Stem cells are responsible for inflammation reaction and the release of histamine in the body.

Usually you use antihistamine against allergies and colds symptoms but not without the risk of side effects.

Chlorella is a natural alternative that does not cause side effects.

Chlorella lowers cholesterol and triglycerides whose levels are determined by liver metabolism as well as fat intake.

L.F. Wang, et al., Effect of Chlorella on the Levels of Glycogen, Triglyceride and Cholesterol in Ethionine-Treated Rats. From Journal of the Formosa Medical Association, Vol 79, No. 1, Jan. 1980, pp. 1-10)

We can see how chlorella's protective and purifying effects on the liver can support the body's own self-defense. A clean and healthy bloodstream, rich in oxygen-bearing red blood cells, provides the basis for strong defense against disease.

Chlorella's cleansing activities on the liver and other organs help maintain healthy and clean blood. Clean and fresh blood effectively removes metabolic waste from cells and tissues.

Building up metabolic waste in less active organs and systems is as dangerous as exposure to air and water poisoning, inadequate nutrition in the diet and chemicals at work-places or at home.

(Effects of Chlorella on the Levels of Cholesterol in Serum and Liver, M. Okuda T. Hasegawa, M. Sonoda T Okabe and Y. Tanaka, Japanese Journal of Nutrition, 33 (1) 3-8, 1975).

At Wakahisa Hospital of Fukuoka In Japan, 5 grams of chlorella was administrated to 16 patients with hyper-cholesterolemia (chronic high blood cholesterol levels), while all other medications and special diets being completed.

Serum cholesterol levels were clearly lowered after three months. The above mentioned effects of chlorella and CGF are only a fraction of the results of experimental and research work carried out over the past 80 years.
In summary, many doctors, physicians, therapists and medical researchers in many countries recommend the use chlorella pyrenoidosa.

Complete: Chlorella is not exposed to any type of refining process. Its entire cell, full with vital nutrients is available to the body.
Pure: Chlorella is not exposed to chemical pesticides or chemicals used in agriculture.
Nor is it added preservatives, artificial colors or flavors or other chemicals.
Natural: As nature created this algae included the persistent and healing factors from the cellular nucleus itself.
Digest ability: The disintegration process used for the chlorella cell has rendered algae digestible to about 80%.
High Chlorophyll content: Chlorella content of chlorophyll (2-7%) is higher than of any other known plant. Chlorophyll is, according to expertise, the most effective cleansing agent for the body's cells.
Nutritious: Chlorella contains 55-65% protein, 20-25% carbo-hydrates, 5-15% fat, of which 82% are unsaturated and 12% saturated fats. Chlorella contains 19% amino acids, including all the essential.
Vitamins: Provitamin A, B1 (thiamine), B2 (riboflavin), B3 (niacin), B6 (pyrodixin), B12, pantothenic acid, folic acid, biotin, PABA, inositol and vitamins C, D and E.

Minerals: Iron, phosphorus, magnesium, calcium, iodine, zinc, potassium, copper, sulfur, manganese, sodium, cobalt and selenium traces.

Normalization of the intestinal tract: Chlorella helps restore an underdeveloped intestinal system to be able to function normally and regularly. **Chlorophyll** in chlorella cleans and removes bad odor from the intestine. Chlorella's cell wall containing sporopollenin (only in chlorella pyrenoidosa) collects and transports toxins, foreign bacterial pesticides and heavy metals from the body.

Intestinal purification: chlorophyll in chlorella helps to purify the blood while iron, vitamin B12 and folic acid help to "build up new red blood cells.

Protection of the liver: Animal experiments show that chlorella helps protect the liver from various poisonous products.

Hypertonia (high blood pressure): Chlorella stimulates to normalizing of too high blood pressure, in many cases after a few months of use. Blood cholesterol and triglycerides have also been reduced by the intake of chlorella.

Growth factor:
Nuclear material in chlorella stimulates cell division, tissue repair, according to research results from Japanese hospitals.

Acidification/Alkaline Balance: Chlorella neutralizes excess acids and heavy acidity in the body as well as maintaining good acid/ alcalins balance.

Immunity: Previous studies show that chlorella enhances the immune system and strengthens the body's own defense mechanism against disease by strengthening at least 5 major factors in the immune system.

Chlorella balances and normalizes metabolism in the body. Chlorella contains the entire vitamin B-complex, vitamin E, D and C, and among minerals there are magnesium, calcium, iron and suitable and necessary to be eaten by everyone, from children to adults regardless of age and very important for pregnant women.

Chlorella is a strong antioxidant and helps the body to build and maintain a strong immune system which today is more necessary than ever, to counteract against cardiovascular disease, viruses, allergies and cancers.

One of the factors that distinguish chlorella from other algae is CGF (chlorella growth factor).

Another factor is the special cell wall that enclosing and protect chlorella's nutritional content and contributing to attracting heavy metals and other foreign substances and bringing these toxins through the intestinal tract.

Chlorella contains most in the world of the so important nutrients chlorophyll and RNA/ DNA!

RNA/DNA are nuclear factors whose growth occurs naturally in our body but as age deteriorates in quality perhaps already from the age of 20 years.

Nutritional power.

The human body is basically capable of curing itself if it receives stimulation and access to necessary vitamins, minerals, enzymes, fatty acids, proteins and other required nutrients. There are, although to a small extent, nutrients in some parts of our daily diet that are useful and may assist the body to maintain good health, but hardly anything with such complete and nutritional content as chlorella.

In addition to its ability to daily detoxify the body from foreign bacteria and heavy metals, Chlorella provides the body with 100% natural, easily absorbable and complete nutrients that are needed to prevent and maintain good health.
For this reason, millions of people around the world are eating chlorella every day of the year as an important supplement to todays food.

When we get a problem, we should first get to know the reason, being a first step of many, to reach the goal to better health.
It is also important to learn about the body's own resources and how to best use them for a faster and better way of solution to the problem.

Only when the problem becomes acute and we feel tired depressed, annoyed or sick, it is important to understand the cause and immediately seek solution for a healthier and better quality of life.

The cause of chronic disease is associated with two processes, the lack of biochemical elements and the accumulation of toxic substances in the body which weakens our natural immune system.
Fatigue, reduced energy and mental depression are the body's signals showing us that we live incorrectly and that we should change our lifestyle.
    Having the knowledge of and the power to set them up correctly, would be something wonderful to look forward to.
One is talking more and more about self-esteem, but it is desirable to eventually achieve good cooperation between school medicine and alternative care.

The first step to reach a better quality of life, is to eat right and healthy food.
We ought to stop to provide our body daily with nutritionally poor food and junk food that adds to they blood toxic sub-stances which adds to the blood, toxic substances and contributes to acidification.
It is so important to think about the pH value and try to create a good acid/base balance in the body.

We should stop providing too much of refined sugar, wheat flour, ready-made and packaged foods, dairy products, coffee, bad tea, fried foods and other types of food that our common sense tells us being far from appropriate, useful and healthy.

It is most important to avoid soft drinks, junk food, candy and other sweets as well as to reduce intake of carbohydrates in the form of potatoes and pastas and in particular bad fats and trans fats.
We should eliminate or reduce our consumption of red meat in our diet, avoid pork meat and use less of unnecessary medicines which are so often used with excessive exaggeration.
Instead, we should use nutritional products from nature in our diet; fresh, complete and "live food".
Eating junk food means acidifying the body and thus increasing the level of poisons which is a major and difficult obstacle in order to obtain good health.

Complete and "Live food" together with exercises, less stress, fresh air, sunshine, recreation, a positive attitude, meaningful work and enough sleep, all together, will give us all a healthier and happier life.

If we do not eat proper food, the immune system hurts the body as well as our different organs and its functions.

Nutritional advice..
Chlorella contains vitamins, minerals, fatty acids, amino acids, chlorophyll and DNA/RNA. Chlorella's total nutritional content is genetically recognized by humans and animals and can thus, be absorbed more quickly and efficiently in the body.
In the the treatment of chlorella pyrenoidosa of best quality, no chemical substances or foreign substances and foreign aids are used.

***Let* your food be your medicine- let your medicine be your food.**
Hippokrates, Greek teacher, "father of medicine" and operating on the island of Kos in the Aegean Sea in the year 460-about 370 BC.

In top form with chlorella
An old saying says that for every disease there is an herb and another one says that you become what you eat! The Chinese and Japanese have since been convinced that chlorella can contribute to a better health balance in the body and give both physical and mental stimulus.
Healthy cells
The human body consists of more than 100 billion cells, most of
which are renewing constantly.
The human body consists of more than 100 billion cells, most of which are renewing constantly.
In the first place, the number of cells are constant during life for each human.

However with aging, cellular functions weakens as well as gradually the number of cells decreases. With the aid of proteins, carbohydrates and fats, the body provides the fuel (calories) as energy supply to our cells. Vitamins and minerals are necessary nutrients by which the intercellular combustion process is started by energy recovery.

If we take up more fuel than the body uses, it is converted to fat and stored as hidden reserves.

A well-balanced nutrition retains the absorption of fuel and vital substances.

Being in biochemically good form means that every body cell is constantly supplied with natural vitamins and minerals and not with overdose of so called empty fuel calories (such as carbohydrates and fats).

The biochemical condition is not to be confused with muscle conditioning.

In order to improve and maintain a better health condition, one should primarily consider and take into account the biochemical condition. In order to improve and maintain a better health condition, one should consider the biochemical condition.

Chlorella is an ideal nutritional supplement for anyone who wishes to improve and maintain good health.

However, in order to obtain a better quality of life, it is important to treat the body as a whole.

Eating the right food and to seek an individualized lifestyle is an important combination. Lifestyle also includes planning your day better which helps to reduce stress.

Of course, it is important to eat at certain times three meals of food every day. Since we consist of 70% to

80% liquid, it is important to drink 1 - 2 liters of water every day. Do not forget the necessity of the daily exercise. You need to jog or run or walk to the gym to keep in good and healthy shape. It works equally well with at least 1 hour of daily walking with changing pace or why not a rod walk that trains the entire body.

Many people who eat chlorella report that they experience increased performance and improved physical and mental fitness already after 4 to 6 weeks. Since all people react differently, it may take 2 to 3 months, taking a daily dose of about 3 grams (l5 tablets), before you notice improvement of the overall health condition. We can not live a healthy life by only trying to replace bad eating habits with good nutritional supplements.

The most important factor is still to use good eating habits if you want to treat yourself well for your good health and preventing diseases. Without eating the right food we can not regain or rejuvenate tissues, nor keep healthy tissues in the body.

All unbalanced nutrition contributes to mineral deficiency somewhere in the body and deficiency of minerals is the first step towards progressive disease.

EATING THE RIGHT FOOD AT THE RIGHT TIME IS TO MAKE YOURSELF A GREAT SERVICE!

CLEANING PROCESS IN THE BODY.
What may be most important for the well-being of the body, is to continuously remove it from heavy metals and other foreign matters.

We know that a body is exposed to pollution from both external (exotoxins) and internal (endorphin) sources every day.

Examples of exotoxins are poisons, industrial chemicals dumped in the nature, chemicals that are supplied to our soils and treated water and industrial emissions due to air pollution.
Endotoxins are bacteria in the body being released from byproducts by the digestive tract which may have a toxic effect when absorbed.

In the case of common digestion, substances that have to be eliminated such as lactic acid, uric acid and more are also produced.

Toxic substances included in the food, everywhere in the environment, in the air we breathe and the water we drink constitute the biggest health problem of each day. They contribute to a variety of our modern illnesses and inconveniences.
More than ever before, we expose ourselves daily to more chemicals, both from those chemically produced and from those that are naturally occurring.

Evan thorough the body has a significant ability to clear these and other poisons, we must constantly stimulate and support it in carrying out this important detoxification process. There is a constant development of new chemicals, maybe even 1000s, which together form an increasingly accelerating danger to us humans and animals.
It is estimated that, to date, there are about 100,000 foreign chemicals such as various pesticides, industrial chemicals, medicines and food additives.
  It's not always easy to defend oneself effectively and sufficiently against smoking, air pollution, amalgam fillings, nutritional supplements (substances in the food, chemicals in drinking water), drugs, vacci-

nations, tattoos, influenza injections, cosmetics chemicals, chemicals absorbed from synthetic textiles in clothing, paints, plastics, pesticides, fertilizers spread on our fields and in our soils, gardens, radiation from medical X-rays, nuclear power stations, computers, cell phones, radios, microwave ovens, power lines, radio and satellite broadcasting.

We know that toxic overload gives us a variety of problems such as depressive disorders, mental blurring, headache, migraine, joint and muscular pain, allergic reactions and cardiac arrhythmia.
We also know that it can lead to more serious conditions, like autoimmune diseases where the symptoms arise from the formation of antibodies directed against the antagonists of the muscles (receptors) for signals from the nerves.
    Example of an autoimmune disease is rheumatoid arthritis. Toxic overload can also lead to neurological diseases such as Parkinson's and Alzheimer's. People suffering from these diseases are considered to be particularly sensitive to poisoning. It is very important that you get right nutrition and that you want to find a good nutrition balance as this is crucial to the body's own ability to eliminate poisons.
Examples of toxic heavy metals for the body are cadmium, arsenic, lead, nickel, mercury (50% in amalgam fillings), uranium and aluminum.
Examples of other foreign poisonous substances are pesticides in food, PCBs (polychlorinated biphenyl), DDT, home-based chemicals such as vinyl chloride and styrene, hydrogenated bad fats from fried and roasted food, alcohol and pharmaceuticals. The heavy metals accumulate in the kidneys, the brain and our immune system whose functions are disturbed.

It is now dependent on the body's own ability to neutralize poisons and remove its own anti-oxidant production.

As far as mercury is concerned, the body has not learned to produce antioxidants against this heavy metal, so it can freely interfere with energetic production on the inside of individual nerve cells.
   This causes the nerve cell's ability to get rid of the poison, causing it to be poisoned and dying with the result that a variety of health problems can occur.
The body's own form of protection against poisonous substances depends largely on the condition of our detoxification, skin, lungs and intestines and their way through the liver and kidneys. Perhaps, nonetheless, the intestines are the main organs of detoxification. They change their ability to release toxins due to nutritional dieting, medication and stress and environ-mental damage. Normally, the intestines release small molecules, but by leaking intestines, large molecules and substances are released into the blood that can cause disease.   These substances affect the entire body and can also be linked to inflammatory joint diseases.
Why a person can have a leaky bowel may be due to chronic nutritional deficiency, bacterial overgrowth as well as imbalances in the intestinal flora.

To help the body protect the intestinal barrier, it is important to:
Restrict the use of anti-inflammatory medicine (may be associated with the formation of small intestine wounds). Minimize the intake of coffee, alcohol and processed foods. Try to manage and cope with stress in an effort to balance the hormonal system.

Chew the food well and make sure your food is well digested. Eat in piece and harmony and strengthen the digestive enzymes.
Add suitable nutrition to the intestines by eating raw vegetables and raw fruit. Be careful to maintain a good micro flora balance in your intestine.

Chlorella as food.
Chlorella contains growth-stimulating substances, making it valuable as an ingredient in bread and fermented beverages.
If Chlorella extract are added to the dough prior to fermentation, both appearance and taste are enhanced while the bread stays fresh for a longer time. Chlorella can also be added to cheese, mayonnaise, pasta and rice to enhance the taste and improve nutritional value.
  Chlorella has an enhancing effect on the body's cells by enhancing our metabolic pathways as well as having an amount of RNA and DNA that can be associated with delayed aging. Nutritionally, chlorella is almost a perfect food. Each small cell is a complete plant with all its attributes intact. It is natural without any additives or by-products as it is cultured in clean environment and is only positively affected by the sun's nutritional light .
  The chlorella plant is natural and without any additives and byproducts, nor does it neglect its nutritional value in cultivation and handling processes. In sealed packaging, it stays as fresh for many years and it contains only 400 to 460 calories per 100 grams. Chlorella's strong and thick cell wall has allowed it to survive for more than 3 billion years on earth, despite

drastic changes in climate and other environmental conditions.

The outer membrane consists of cellulose which is difficult to digest for humans and therefore caused many comments by scientists who examined chlorella in the 1950s. Many scientific attempts were made to make chlorella more accessible and absorbable to the human body in order to use it as a nutritious food.

The first and best method patented by a Japanese company was created in the late 1970s, which resulted in that chlorella became easier to digest to about 80%. Thus, chlorella's nutritional properties were more accessible to humans and could therefore be utilized better as healthy food.

Today only only a few accepted methods exist to powder chlorella's strong cell wall. The famous nutritionist, Dr. Bernard Jensen explained that **"it's not what we eat that matters but what our body can absorb from the nutrition we eat."** It is a fact that a good quality of chlorella is being absorbable to 80% which means that a significantly higher percentage of its nutrients, can be absorbed by the blood from the small intestine. Interestingly, fish, chicken and meat consist of between 20% to 30% protein, while 80% of fish protein is used by the body, and about 67% chicken and meat protein is used. Chlorella is thus one of the most easily digestible and absorbable proteins I know.

Nowadays, chlorella has proved to be a potentially functional diet, not only for those who eat an unbalanced, low nutritional and environmental impacted diet, but could instead be able to contribute to a potential solution for a world of starving and which handicap many of poor nations on earth.

Few nutritions have gained such scientific attention in so many countries and in as short a time as chlorella especially during a time when it appears that the nutritional reserves of the world are becoming increasingly depleted and perhaps soon will reach a dangerous level.

Soils in many countries are already overworked and exhausted on important and necessary nutrients that you can no longer grow nutritional crops.

Finally, the result is that depleted soils produce depleted crops, depleted crops create depleted people and exhausted body functions create diseases. Unlike most crops, chlorella is grown in water and not in the soil. Chlorella transforms organic and inorganic chemicals into active, live, organic food with existing solar energy to give the body vitalizing food that it can fully utilize. It is likely that, one of chlorella's main contributions, is its ability to balance body chemistry. Although nutrition knowledge is now being applied more than 40 years ago, it has not been possible to maintain the same good nutritional basis, but it is in imbalance in most countries through continued cultural traditions that emphasize specific food.

Research reports from the world
Chlorella pyrenoidosa is probably the most carefully researched food in our time with thousands of research papers published over the years from several medical universities in the world. Documents show chlorella's versatile ability to stimulate the body for better balance and thus to a better health in a variety of cases.

This primarily demonstrates chlorella's overall beneficial effects, but I think it is important for readers to participate in a more detailed technical discussion.

The healing properties of chlorella pyrenoidosa have been documented since many years, in Japan among other places. Japanese clinical studies and reports have shown and proven chlorella's beneficial role in the treatment of a number of chronic diseases including various forms of cancer.

As mentioned earlier, we are exposed daily to environmental pollutants in air, water (also drinking water) and food. From fields and cultivation, millions of tonnes of toxic waste from pesticides leak into groundwater. We are exposed to heavy metals in dental care and from toxins through overuse of drugs.

We are exposed to radiation from cell phones, microwave ovens, and televisions that can cause radiation damage. Symptoms are suggesting that this could be cancer, leukemia, poor thyroid function, severe hair loss, loss of appetite, insomnia, infertility, impotence, concentrating difficulty and poor blood values.

Due to poor oral hygiene with hidden toxins in our teeth as a result, many diseases develop and, in particular, the body is subjected to toxins due to pronged mental stress.

These toxins cause us to more quickly grow older by breaking down our immune system and health.

It is estimated for example, that there are more than 80000 different synthetic chemicals from air pollution and industrial emissions that contribute to our body acidification.

These environmental hazards and pollutants affect our body systems including cells, glands, intestines, lungs, nervous system, liver and lymphatic system.

The central nervous system is most sensitive to poison in the blood stream.

DETOXIFICATION FROM ENVIRONMENTAL HAZARDS

Chlorella is used to detoxify persons suffering from the effects of PCB poisoning.
Dr Useda from Kitakyushu City Institute for Environmental Pollution Research in Japan, gave during a year, 6 grams daily of chlorella to 30 patients exposed to PCB poisoning. The result was an almost 100% improvement in patients (less fatigue, better digestion, normal bowel movement).

In 1984, Drug and Chemical Toxicology published a study by Dr Pore at West Virginia University, the School of Medicine, in which chlorella administrated to rats could strengthen the detoxification effects against hydrocarbon chlorine's toxic and harmful insecticides. It was found that chlorella contributed to the removal of the toxin from the body more than 2 times faster than in the control group.
Dr Pore found two active absorbent mechanisms of chlorella: sporopollenin, a carotene-like polymer and the cell wall itself.

DETOXIFICATION OF HEAVY METALS.

Cadmium poisoning is a price we must pay to live in a modern industrialized world. High doses of cadmium have been associated with high blood pressure in animated studies.

According to researchers at Memorial University, Newfoundland St. Johns in Canada, cadmium is a toxic heavy metal more or less most people are exposed to.

As a newborn, there is no cadmium in the tissues but this heavy metal accumulates for a lifetime and accumulates in considerable amounts in the average human.

The source of exposure to cadmium for most people includes pollutants from food and smoking.
In addition people employed in the manufacturing industry are exposed using cadmium or other bypro-ducts, as this heavy metal is in alloying, paint manufacturing, plastics and cadmium nickel batteries, melting and refining of zinc and lead.
    Smoking reduces the ability of the blood to deliver oxygen to the heart which reduces the potential of this vital organ to create energy molecules.
Smoking also increases the blood clotting activity of the cells that can block blood flow and destroy the arteries by supporting the formation of coronary artery injury and coronary disease. Russian researchers found that cadmium, alongside other heavy metals, are involved in the activation of blood clot formation.
    It was suspected that the cadmium also contributes to high blood pressure and arteriosclerosis.
 In 1975, a Japanese scientist Hagino et al. said that chlorella increased excretion of cadmium in individuals suffering from cadmium poisoning.
Thanks to chlorella's ability to bind to cadmium, re-searchers wanted to ensure that, as soon as the cad-mium was bound to chlorella, it would not be able to return to the body.
It was found that chlorella could attract cadmium and other heavy metals, to retain them and then bring them through the intestinal system and it has also been shown that zinc helps prevent degradation of the

immune system caused by cadmium poisoning among others due to tobacco smoking.

Other studies have shown the ability of chlorella pyrenoidosa to bind also other heavy metals and poisons like mercury, copper, uranium and lead, DDT and PCBs and remove them out of the body.

FIBROMYALGIA

Fibromyalgia is a syndrome associated with diminishing nightly secretion of melatonin. Fibromyalgia is a chronic condition with muscular aches characterized by pain sensation in the muscles of the skeleton, tendons (muscular stress) and ligaments throughout the body. Other symptoms may be depression, stiffness fatigue and sleep disorders.

Typically, tenderness is in the 11-19 trigger points. Common pain areas are lower back, shoulders, arms and knees. In stress, these pains are exacerbated as well as in weather conditions.

Depression usually occurs in fibromyalgia as well as mood swings, numbness, stomach ache, swollen fingers, irritated mucous membranes and often dizziness.

The problem can lead to decreased immune system and intestinal infections.

Curing fibromyalgia can be difficult but good chances are if you change your lifestyle, which in many cases, have resulted in full recovery. Eating the right food, exercise, having good sleep (deep enough), positive thinking and, not least, the addition of important nutrition.

It is of utmost importance to daily detoxify the body from heavy metals and other toxins that can fundamentally be contributing causes of fibromyalgia.

10 g of Chlorella taken daily for 2 months was associated with a 22 % decrease in pain (assessed by TPI)
in one pilot study in 18 persons with Fibromyalgia.

Double blind, placebo-controlled and randomized
clinical trials were performed on 55 people with
fibromyalgia, 33 with elevated blood pressure, 9
people with ulcerative colitis. Patients receive 10
grams of pure chlorella pyrenoidosa in tablet form and
100 ml of CGF (chlorella water extract) daily for two
months.
The result clearly demonstrated the decrease in blood
pressure and serum cholesterol levels, accelerated
wound healing, and improved immune functions as
well as relief of the above symptoms.

In the above as also in other trials, the conclusion
was that chlorella could alleviate symptoms, improve
quality of life and normalize body functions in patients
with fibromyalgia, high blood pressure and ulcerative
colitis.

(Source: RE Merchant and CA. Other, "A Review of Recent
Clinical Trials of the Nutritional Supplement Chlorella
Pyrenoidosa in the Treatment of Fibromyalgia, Hypertension
and Ulcerative Colitis," Alternative Therapies in Health and
Medicine 7 No. 3, May, June 2001)

Chlorella brings down cholesterol levels.
Chlorella can diminish hypercholesterolemia according
to scientific studies. Only a very small percentage of
cholesterol level from food is presented in our blood. It
is the human body itself that produces the cholesterol.
Cholesterol is necessary for the body (<120mg%) and
an insufficient level, is as dangerous as a too high
cholesterol level.

Pulmonary arteries

Pulmonary artery

Left atrium

Superior vena cava

His' bundle

Right atrium

Left ventricle

Sinoatrial node
Atrioventricular node

Orifice of inferior vena cava

Left branch of AV bundle

Right ventricle

Right branch of AV bundle

R

T

P

U

0.1 sec.
0.2 sec.

O

S

0.08 - 0.1 sec.

Ventricular muscle
contraction

Ventricular relaxation
(repolarization)

Intra-atrial transmission

Atrioventricular His   Intraventricular transmission

CHLORELLA AND THE HEART

High serum cholesterol concentrations are major risk
factors for cardiac disease. A daily intake of 5 grams of
Chlorella was associated with significant reductions in
problems of heart health and it increases in carotenoids, according to findings.
Daily consumption of chlorella, provide the potential of
health benefits reducing serum lipid risk factors like
triglycerides and total cholesterol mildly hyper-
cholesterolemia subjects.

Regular consumptions of Chlorella supplement (5 g/day) over 4 weeks significantly reduced serum triglyceride, total cholesterol, non-HDL-cholesterol, LDL-cholesterol, [the ratio of HDL- cholesterol to triglycerides], and Apo B (Apo lipoprotein B) in subjects with mild hyper-cholesterolaemia.

A study shows that daily consumption of Chlorella supplement resulted in significant increases in serum lutein/zeaxanthin and alpha carotene concentrations.
Chlorella contains a relatively high percentage of omega-3 fatty acids, which is known not to inhibit chylomicron assembly in the intestine, but to inhibit LDL assembly in the liver.
Chlorella is a good source of dietary fiber that affects lymphatic cholesterol and triglyceride absorption by increasing gut viscosity, altering the composition of the bile acid pool, and also producing fermentation products in the intestine.

Researchers believe that chlorella can reduce side effects from chemotherapy and show "anti-tumor activity".
In 1996, a report was published in the journal Cancer Immunology and Immunotherapy" about clinical activity of chlorella against side effects in the treatment of cancer drug 5-Flouracil (5FU). The side effects include leukopenia (abnormally large number of white blood cells) which can result in infections.

The researchers found that extracts of chlorella, not only prevented the adverse reaction of 5FU, but also demonstrated direct anti-cancer activity. The researchers considered that the anti-cancer effect depends on chlorella's ability to stimulate T-cell activity.

In 1995, "Phytochemistry" published a study conducted by Japanese researchers who identified and isolated two glyceroglycolipids with anti-tumor ability. According to the researchers' description, two elements in chlorella had been shown to possess inhibitory activity against a foreign protein associated with Epstein-Barr virus.

In 1984, **Cancer Immunology and Immunotherapy** published a study entitled "The Department of immunology" at the Medical Institute of Bioregulation, Yushu University (Japan). It was found that "the growth of Meth-A tumor in mice was clearly inhibited by injection of CGF into the tumor or in tissues surrounding the tumor itself" In addition, the mice treated with CGF antigen, specifically demonstrated increased resistance to continued tumor formation.

Chlorophyll content of Chlorella pyrenoidosa
Chlorella pyrenoidosa contains more chlorophyll (minimum 28.9 g / kg) than any other plant on earth. (Merchant R and Andre C, 2001. "Dietary supplementation with Chlorella pyrenoidosa produces positive results in patients with cancer or suffering from certain common chronic diseases. JANA 412:31-8)

Chlorophyll and its derivatives form molecular complexes with environmental poisons and disable them by preventing them from binding to DNA and cell receptors. Chlorophyll can also unspecified prevent cytochrome P450 activity by reducing phase I molecular processes that can lead to cancerous activation.

Researchers believe that chlorophyll works primarily by inhibiting Phase I cytochrome P450 enzymatic channel (an important detoxification channel in the body, found in almost all cells) responsible for the activation of cancerous toxins. Researchers at Shapporo Medical University, supported an analysis (in vitro) performed with chlorella pyrenoidosa in conjunction with detoxification processes, which showed that consumption of 4 to 5 grams of chlorella before varying amounts of alcohol was consumed, resulted in a 96% decrease in reaction of "hangover".

This finding shows that chlorella strengthens the liver detoxification capacity by facilitating the removal of alcohol from the liver (Steenblock D. "Chlorella, Natural Medicinal Algae." Aging Research Institute, CA, US, 1987).

In addition to chlorella's proven amount of chlorophyll that successfully binds and supports the deposition of environmental pollutants, this single-cell algae contains additional properties that work synergistically with chlorophyll improving the liver's detoxification channels. It is important to note that chlorella also contains glutathione, a key component by phase II detoxification of the liver. Glutathione is important both as an antioxidant and as functional conjugation group in Phase II.
 Glutathione occurs in Chlorella growth factor (CGF) a complex of nutritional and functional components that demonstrate a variety of medical properties.

Why is it good to eat chlorella?
Chlorella is a good nutrition, that is to say, it is a food that contain nutrients that can assist and stimulate a

better body balance and reinforcement for our so vital organs. Unfortunately, you do not find enough of this full nutritional content in your daily normal diet.

Fully nutrient means raw food (live food) that contains easily absorbable and well balanced, complete nutrition in 100% organic natural forms.

***We can call it living food or functional food**.*
Vegetables and fruits in raw form, not cooked or fried or otherwise processed so that their nutritional content is damaged (enzyme loss) are also live foods and functional foods. Certainly these, basically good and healthy nutrients, are treated with spraying, it is better to eat raw vegetables and fruits rather than completely exclude them from the diet. Today it's hard to find raw substances that have not been treated in any way, but fortunately there are now organic-grown vegetables and fruits for those who wish. Although it seems more expensive to buy organic farmed vegetables, it may still be worth the price many times.

* You can carefully wash both vegetables and fruits in water added with a few drops of apple cider vinegar and let them lie in the water for about half an hour before rinsing.
* It is not advisable to prepare vegetables and fruit by boiling or roasting them if you want to benefit from the nutritional content. When heated up to about 45 degrees, enzymes disappear largely, which is negative because we need these for our digestion.
* It is also worth noting that lycopene in tomatoes, which is also beneficial against the risk of prostate cancer, is more efficiently extracted when the tomatoes are heated before ingestion.

* Separate the shell from the tomato after a short warming up as this is difficult to digest.
* Likewise, it is advantageous to steam boil carrots to let the beta carotene rise although it also increases the carbohydrates in the carrot when heated.
* A good general tip is to always eat a salad before the intake of protein-rich foods like meat because the vegetables form a good enzyme basis for better combustion.

QUESTIONS AND ANSWERS

Q: What is CHLORELLA pyrenoidosa?
A: Chlorella is a microscopic green freshwater plant with a true cell nucleus. Chlorella's single cell structure has a rich content of concentrated vitamins, minerals, protein and other nutrients. Thanks to that chlorella is a clean, complete and balanced nutrition, this alga is perfectly suited to be consumed by both humans and animals (100% natural vegetable). Chlorella has more than 50 different vitamins and minerals and provides us with lots of natural beta-carotene. Chlorella is 60% to 70% proteins and has the largest amount of chlorophyll of all plants on earth.

Chlorella is rich of iron, calcium, potassium, phosphorus, magnesium, zinc, copper, traces of selenium, sulphur and cobalt, and 19 amino acids of which the 8 essential. **Chlorella contains more vitamin B12 than is found in beef liver.** This vitamin is otherwise, often missing in other vegetarian food.

Q: HOW DOES CHLORELLA WORK?
A: Combination of Chlorella's special cell wall with sporopollenin (only occurs in Chlorella pyrenoidosa) and the large amount of chlorophyll, as well as some

of the important proteins in chlorella, attract heavy metals, such as mercury, lead, copper, cadmium, palladium and uranium that are effectively removed through the intestines.

The same applies to solvents, PCBs, DDT, alcohol, nicotine, dioxin and other toxins. In many of the worlds' countries, chlorella has been used for a long time in connection with the remediation of amalgam/ mercury. The synergy effect of the large amount of nutrition in Chlorella helps the balance and stabilize processes on the cell level in our body. Chlorella provides the body with nutrition and opportunities for remediation from toxins in order to function with maximum capacity and efficiency.

With this as a background and on a daily basis, Chlorella acts as an "upload". Millions of people eat chlorella every day for the purpose of preventing disease and maintaining good health.

Q. CAN CHLORELLA HELP ME LOSE OR INCREASE IN WEIGHT?

A: Chlorella is no dietary food but is a balanced and complete nutritional food.

Many people claim that they are getting better energy and the sweets requirement decreases when eating chlorella. This is especially true for people who use other types of weight loss programs.

As a complete diet with 60-70% protein chlorella still contains only 12 calories in a daily dose of 3 grams or 15 tablets. Chlorella satisfies the appetite while providing good nutrition that gives us energy.

Not least important, when trying to lose weight, is to stop consuming too much of sugar and unnecessary bad fat and to consume the body's need for essential fatty acids.

Chlorella is very rich in essential fatty acids, among others (Omega-3 and omega-6).
Chlorella helps in digestion, metabolism and contributes to more efficient emptying of the bowel. This results in a better absorption and burning of the food you eat. Chlorella's ability to detoxify the body and to normalize acid/base balance also contributes to prevent weight gain.
Whether the goal is to reduce or increase weight, Chlorella can help balance the body's functions which in turn leads to a more permanent change of your health and weight. Chlorella in tablet or powder form taken in conjunction with the meal, can also in many cases give some sense of saturation.

Chlorella is also known as an adaptogen (substance that generally strengthens the immune system) which makes it easier to cope with stress factors and defend us against external bacterial attacks. Adaptogens reduces hormones associated with stress. These stress hormones have a number of negative effects on the body that can make us to eat more but cause poorer digestion, which together leads to weight gain.
As an adaptogen, chlorella lowers production of stress hormones which contributes to better control of appetite and improvement of digestion.

Q: IS CHLORELLA A SUBSTITUTE FOR OTHER VITAMINS AND MINERAL SUPPLEMENTS?

A: We recommend chlorella as a supplement to the daily diet, which usually lacks sufficient nutrition.
Chlorella contains a more balanced, complete and body efficient nutrition in natural form as synthetically produced products are missing real nutrients and multivitamins.

In addition chlorella contains a number of other nutrients and substances with functions that cannot be found in synthetic nutritional supplements, among others, chlorophyll, RNA/DNA, albumin, xanthophyll.

Chlorella is "Functional Food".
Many so called "natural" vitamins and minerals are manufactured by foreign substances, foreign to the body, such as coal, tar products, animal by-products/ waste and excrement, ground stones, shells and metals). For example vitamin B12 (cyanocobalamin) may be made from toxic residues of cow liver or sewage sludge.
Vitamin A comes from fish liver oil filled with toxic PCBs and mercury, B vitamins from carbon, tar and petrochemicals, known to weaken the nervous system, give depression, irritation to the respiratory system and is cancerous.

Chlorella pyrenoidosa, on the other hand, is grown under the strictest control, treated and packaged under certified forms in the case of recognized and documented chlorella products.

Q: IS CHLORELLA BENEFICIAL TO EAT WHEN BODY BUILDING?
A: Absolutely. The nucleic acids in chlorella have contributed to the fact that this plant reproduces itself at very high speed.
When we eat chlorella we also eat the nucleic acids that are responsible for chlorella's rapid cell repro- duction along with all the nutrition that occurs in chlorella's reproductive growth and maintenance of its life span.

The nucleic acids in chlorella regulate the body's production of enzymes, proteins and energy. These nucleic acids also help the body to use meat proteins by converting them to amino acids that in turn converts into proteins according to RNA and DNA specifications. If you eat Chlorella in conjunction with protein powder chlorella can induce a synergistic effect. Chlorella is low-calorie, and contains only a small amount of sodium, which is why this alga is suited to today's bodybuilders and their lifestyle

Q: What is the difference between CHLORELLA, ALFALFA, SPIRULINA and SPROUTS.

A: Many "green" foods are sources of chlorophyll which is important. However in comparison, chlorella contains most chlorophyll of all known plants. Microbiologists who recently conducted laboratory tests, point to that chlorella contains 3-5 times more chlorophyll than spirulina, another nutritional organism albeit somewhat more primitive than chlorella.

Spirulina is a more primitive organism and a cyanogen bacteria, because this alga lacks a true nucleus, meaning that chlorella with a true nucleus has a higher quality of RNA and DNA and is a real plant.

Chlorella also supplies us with more iron and essential fatty acids than spirulina. Spirulina lacks vitamin C.

Chlorella also contains 15 - 20 times more chlorophyll than alfalfa. In fact, 2%-7% of chlorella is chlorophyll, the largest content among all known plants in the world. Chlorella gives us the advantage of having access to all the protoplasts that help in the growth, development and repair of our own cells! Chlorella is alone in containing CGF (Chlorella Growth Factor).

Q: WHAT IS CGF.
A: CGF is a concentrated hot water extract of chlorella's cell nucleus. CGF contains nucleic peptides (growth hormones) that are important for development of our own RNA/DNA.

Many nutritionists believe that the natural quality of the body's nucleic acids (RNA/DNA) is rapidly deteriorated by external influences such as contamination, unilateral and unbalanced diet, stress and lack of exercise, lack of good and enough sleep, all of which result in less efficient metabolism and premature aging. Not least, it is important to understand that the body's own production and quality of RNA and DNA is naturally reduced after 20 years of age, when our bodies reach maturity.

CGF (Chlorella Growth Factor) is one of the primary and most important sources of RNA/DNA that contributes to the repair and promotion of our own cells. Chlorella contains 2,5-OD/l/g of CGF.

Q: How much chlorella can I eat?
A: Because chlorella is complete food, one can eat a larger number of tablets daily without risk.

When you begin to eat chlorella, it is good to daily take 1 to 3 pills (especially for people with particularly sensitive intestinal systems) during the first week. This is because the body is to be used to an initial detoxification process.

After a week, the body, is to be used to chlorella's cleansing and detoxifying effects and you can then increase the dose of at least 10 tablets (2 grams). From the third week it is recommended that you take at least 15 tablets (3) grams each day, either for breakfast or divided during the day.

In case of urgent need for extra nutrition, you can increase the dose depending of your wishes or being recommended to.

There are people, especially over 40 years of age, who have developed a thick mucous lining on the small intestinal wall that can interfere with the digestion and the assimilation as well as peristalsis. That is why it could be advisable to eat chlorella pyrenoidosa as it means you go through a special bowel-cleansing program to get rid of the mucus.

Q: Can kids eat chlorella?
A: Absolutely and advantageously. Children from 2-15 years of age can eat the number of tablets corresponding to their age daily. It is especially important for children of school age to eat a good, and balanced amount of essential fatty acids.

A proper balance of these fatty acids can reduce the problems of dyslexia, vapor and other disorders associated with poorer concentration. The so often occurring hyperactivity among children as in adults can also be remedied with a balanced addition of essential fatty acids.

The body needs both omega 3 and omega 6, and both are abundant in chlorella.

Q: Can a becoming mother eat chlorella during pregnancy and when nursing her baby?
A: When a woman becomes pregnant, her body begins to produce extra blood for a developing fetus. Pregnant women are advised to supplement with iron, folate and vitamin B12 during pregnancy to achieve better red blood cell count and nutrition levels.

Low levels of these vitamins and minerals are what make pregnant women feel weak and tired as her body begins accommodation of the new baby inside.

In order to see the beneficial effects of nutrition for pregnant women, researchers gave a group of pregnant Japanese women chlorella supplements.

The large quantity of foliate, iron and vitamin B12 in the chlorella was to improve anaemic conditions in the pregnant women who were given 6 grams of chlorella daily for seven weeks during a gestation period between the 12th and 18th weeks.

In the second and third trimesters, proportions of anaemia, measured by haemoglobin levels, were significantly lower. The proportion of women with edema was also significantly lower in the chlorella-group. Heart and kidney function was better overall and the urine protein level was in a normal state.

Conclusions were stating that "Chlorella supplementation significantly reduces the risk of pregnancy associated anaemia, proteinuria, and edema."

Furthermore, chlorella is "a useful resource of natural foliate, vitamin B12 and iron for pregnant women."

Women seeking a healthy pregnancy should consider clean chlorella as a source of healthy nutrition for them and their baby.

One answer for low iron, folate, and vitamin B12 levels is to use a chlorella supplementation.

This green algae is perfect for pregnant women, welcoming blood-building, vascular strengthening whole food nutritional powers. As natural and complete food, chlorella is important and completely safe for pregnant women who lack nutrition through the diet and often require extra nutritional supplement.

For pregnant woman, it is very important, to every day get rid of toxins from bad food and toxins from the environment, partly for her and partly for the fetus. Researches have showed that also the mother's milk, the baby food, is being cleaned from heavy metals and other toxins when the becoming mother is eating chlorella pyrenoidosa.

Rapid growth of the child requires a lot of protein, vitamins and minerals.

Lack of these substances, can cause permanent damage. Pregnant and breastfeeding women are recommended high protein intake by as much as 70%, but by calories not more than 15%.

The most interesting thing in is that also the greatest food in the world, being mother's own milk to the foster, is cleaned from toxins like heavy metals and foreign bacteria.

At the same time both mother and fetus will assimilate all necessary nutrients from the chlorella pyrenoidosa according to experiences and research.

It is also suggested that during pregnancy, increased intake of the vitamin B complex i necessary.

Chlorella pyrenoidosa is low-calorie food, protein rich and through its concentrate of B-vitamins and other essential nutrients, completely natural and without additives and is of great benefit as a meal supplement, before, during and after pregnancy.

Q: When do you notice effects by eating CHLORELLA?
A: Many people start feeling better and more energetic after a few weeks. Others notice a more clear change for the better after a longer period (2-3 months).

It all depends on the person's individual life style and general physical and mental conditions. However, the best results provide a continuous daily intake, and many say their health situation is getting better the longer they eat chlorella. For more than 110 years, a large number of scientists, nutritionists and doctors in Japan, USA, China and many other countries have researched chlorella.

In particular, it has been emphasized the importance of chlorella's properties to be able to purify kidneys, liver, the intestinal systems and blood using its unique cell wall.

Chlorella attracts foreign substances and heavy metals, being harmful to the body, and expels them through the intestinal tract.

The well-known ability of Chlorophyll to clean and detoxify the body is very important.

Chlorella's contribution to helping the body to get better balance through detoxification and supplements of necessary nutrients, means boosting our immune system, to counteract also genetic diseases and conditions such as cancer, allergies and others.

Q: IS IT IMPORTANT WITH EXTRA NUTRITION FOR WOMEN WITH HEALTH PROBLEMS AND CONDITIONS SUCH AS PMS, OSTEOPOROSIS AND FIBROMYALGIA!
A: Chlorella is a 100% natural product and is normalizing body functions (adaption).
Chlorella is completely non-toxic, easy to use, non-addictive,
100% natural and unlike most drugs, chlorella gives no side effects. Chlorella regulates biological pathways instead of just suppressing symptoms.

PMS e.g. can be reduced by the intake of supplemental vitamin B6 (pyridoxine) that can reduce tension and fluid retention.

On the whole, it is important to think about what you eat, not only just before menstruation, but also always.

If you consider PMS as well as similar disorders that can cause pain, these signs show that the body is out of balance.

Multivitamins and minerals, in natural form as in Chlorella pyrenoidosa, can help to regain the right balance. Women who is experiencing intense pain often have higher levels of prostaglandin, a hormone like substance.

Another cause may also be poor circulation to the uterine muscle. Copper and zinc are important among trace elements.

Vitamin B is an effective hormone regulator and magnesium is also recommended. When a woman gets an improved circulation, she feels less pain along with having less construction of negative prostaglandins. Uneven circulation increases blood loss resulting in loss of iron which leads to anaemia.

Chlorella effectively provides the body with the nutrients it needs in the above mentioned complaints. In order to alleviate and prevent classified issues, it is important to have a good metabolism, to eat the right and balanced food, drink enough of water, to stress less and take care detoxifying the body from foreign substances such as chemicals and heavy metals.

Not least it should be considered to exercise regularly.

When it comes to living healthy and to bring satisfactory nutrition, chlorella can be helpful as this algae is not only rich in nutrition but also that this nutrition is absorbed efficiently in the blood and, inter alia, regulates calcium and iron through its rich content of chlorophyll which also helps to cleanse the body from toxins and is easily assimilated in the same time.

Q: Can I eat CHLORELLA although I use medications?
A: Yes, chlorella has the important characteristic of being able to detoxify the body from foreign substances and thus can help to prevent certain side effects that drugs can cause.

Q: I'm a vegetarian. WHAT CAN CHLORELLA DO FOR ME?
A: Chlorella is rich in proteins and vegetable nutrients. In strict vegetarian diet, chlorella can outweigh the lack of vitamin B and proteins. This applies particularly to vitamin B12.

Q: WHAT CAN CHLORELLA DO BY STOMACH PROBLEMS?
A: Chronic constipation is a major problem as it helps the body collecting toxins and heavy metals that contribute to both obesity, allergies and other diseases. Not least older people suffer from an inconvenience.

In addition to hard stools, constipation also means that those affected suffer from bleeding, bad breath, and reduced blood sugar levels.

It is therefore very important that effective gastro-intestinal emptying can take place one to two times a day.

Scientific studies and investigations show that chlorella seems to stimulate bowel movements (peristalsis), partly because of its high levels of chlorophyll and partly through its detoxifying activity in the intestinal environment.

The intake of chlorella, affects the bowel functions and leads to a more regular and complete emptying of the intestinal tract.

Chlorella stimulates and enhances the effect of the friendly bacteria in the intestine. Remember to drink at least two liters of water every day! Chlorella can be combined with other foods as noodles, bread, soups and other food products.

Perhaps the most interesting is the combination with lactobacillus acidophilus that is bacteria that one normally use to make yogurt.

Scientists found out that adding a little chlorella to the growth medium greatly increases the growth rate of the lactobacillus.

Q: What other health-promoting properties can you expected by eating chlorella?

A: Chlorella is best known as food supplement and as such for its rich composition of photochemical that support the body's natural selfdefense mechanism.

Chlorella detoxifies and supplies the body with nutrition that can help a person to a longer life with good health.

It is logical that when your body is tired, when you are feeling down and tired and undernourished or if any part of your body has a weak point, this part is likely to suffer and with proper and nutritional support, these problems can be remedied.

Chlorella is no miracle cure. The human body as it was created is a miracle by being able to heal itself if it receives a proper and nutritional support.

Over the years, there have been a number of testi-
monies on chlorella's beneficial properties as functional
food. The list of chlorella's good properties is long although many of them are not scientifically investigated.
However, they can still have a physiological explanation, taking into account the basic characteristics
that chlorella has, such as nutritional contents, rejuvenating effects etc.

Chlorella pyrenoidosa

Increase energy and stamina.
Prevent ulcers and eliminate constipation and other
intestinal stomach problems.
Reduce chronic fatigue
Reduce nerve pain
Reduce problems by fibromyalgia.
Reduce allergic reactions
Lowering blood pressure.
Help control diabetes
Check your blood sugar.
Support immune functions.
Reduce rheumatism.
Improve chronic conditions.
Promoting alkaline system.
Regulate appetite.
Reduce appetite.
Reduce cold conditions.
Reduce candida.
Prevent circulation problems, lower cholesterol.
Improve sleep.
Relieve pain
Reduce headache
Reduce diarrhea.
Reduce fertility problems

Reduce Hair Loss.
Reduce athlete problems.
Sharpness memory.
Improves wound healing.
Detoxifying the body.
Decrease heavy metals in the body.
Remove grease.
Prevent "hangover".
Reduce rigidities, PMS Internal bleeding.
Eliminate bad breath.
Heal hemorrhoids.
Increase lifetime living with good health.
Promote liver health.

Chlorella pyrenoidosa contains all the components that are important to a healthy life, making it the most potent food on Earth. Chlorella works for the body's balance and to help to give everyone assistance to lead a healthy life, making it the most nutritionally potent food on earth.

The main activities are to detoxify our body. Toxins cause diseases, imbalances and are harmful for our body. Chlorella pyrenoidosa is a complete, 100 % natural, clean and above all, easily assimilated and useful as a nutrient food product.

Q: Safety and side effects?

A: Chlorella can be safely eaten by adults, elderly, adolescents, pregnant women and nursing mothers without giving side effects. Chlorella can be mixed in soy or oat milk to children who have no access to breast milk or are allergic to cow's milk or milk formula.

In fact, chlorella is far superior to cow's milk that can not provide the body with essential fatty acids which are essential for the optimal development of the immune system, heart, eyes and brain.

As a complete food, chlorella can be eaten in high doses without causing side effects. There has been no harmful effect on children and adults who have been eating chlorella of the highest quality.

After a time of use, beginning the first weeks eating a smaller dose, the body is used to the detoxification process, you can eat large amounts of chlorella.

There is no danger of overdose when taking large amounts of chlorella. Due to chlorella's natural properties to detoxify cells and tissues from toxins, one can experience the following initial reactions in people with strong intestinal poisoning.

1. Gas formation may increase due to increased effect of bowel movements. This reaction decreases as the intestines are purified.

2. In some people although, although in few a certain feeling of nausea can occur for 2 to 3 days.
This feeling is because the body is heavily poisoned and in action to detoxify it from heavy metals.

3. Since the skin is also a cleansing device, some people may temporarily develop acne, rashes, itching or eczema, which is a sign of the body's attempt to regain inner balance while it is working to bring out toxins. It is individual how to react during the first period eating chlorella.
Most people get no clear reactions, and for those who know them, it usually takes 2-5 days for the body to get used to the detoxification process.

If the discomfort still exist after all, it is recommended to halve the proposed dose for a further week or two. Then you can increase the dose as recommended.

Q: How should I use chlorella?
A: It is generally recommended that you take three grams of chlorella every day. One can say that it is for a normally healthy person being the daily need for maintenance. If you take Chlorella to seek relief from any symptoms, double dosage is recommended i.e. 6 grams per day.

Athletes or people who need to exert their body to the utmost, can eat 10 grams or more each day. Because chlorella is a complete diet, it can be eaten at any time with or without other food.

However, it may be an advantage to take chlorella just before other meals because you achieve good help to digest other food.

Chlorella is present in tablet or powder form. CGF (Chlorella Growth Factor) is a hot water extract of chlorella and actually the real nuclear fuel in the algae. Chlorella powder is mixed in a glass of water, fruit or vegetable juice. Mix 1-2 teaspoons of chlorella powder in a glass of water, juice or yogurt and mix well. 1 teaspoon of powder contains about 3 grams of chlorella. In particularly Japan, chlorella powder is often used as an additive in soup, bread, fruit juice, noodles, honey, syrup and tea.

Chlorella is also excellent for fasting as it provides the body with complete natural nutrition, while it also is effectively contributing to detoxification.

Q: Which chlorella products should I choose?
A: There are several different grades of chlorella in the market which are determined by different methods in treating it in cultivation, harvesting and, not least, in the process of making it easily assimilated to humans. Chlorella pyrenoidosa is considered by science to be the most nutritious of other varieties of this algae.

Various methods exist to make chlorella's cell wall digestible and I recommend a method in which the cell wall is crushed or processed so that about 79- 80% of the algae can be effectively utilized by man while maintaining its nutrition.
Today some certain suppliers use "spray drying" under high pressure of chlorella, which is advantageous. Then the nutrient is retained in the cell nucleus while man can easily digest it.
One should choose a chlorella product, which is grown in outdoor pools with clean and mineral-rich water and in areas where there are many sunny days of the year.
In Taiwan and Japan, cultures of chlorella have been in existence for many years where the staff have exten- sive experience and knowledge in treating chlorella. Keep in mind, that chlorella which is grown in indoors tanks does not have the same concentration of important substances as CGF, chlorophyll and protein occurring in chlorella grown in outdoor pools in high- lying areas. This also applies to the content of calcium, iron and vitamins. Natural sunlight can not be replaced by no artificial light, created by man.
Chlorella tablets/powders containing tablet excipients, preservatives, foreign substances, colorants, gluten or other synthetic substances, should **not** be used.

CONCLUSION

Chlorella is a natural and complete diet. From a nutritional point of view, it has an extensive range of nutrients that can stimulate the body's different organs for better functional balance and thus provide a useful tool for prevention and treatment of self-esteem.

From a medical point of view, it has long been demonstrated and proven that this alga detoxifies and strengthens the immune system.

From a clinical point of view, reports show that chlorella is a good aid in the treatment of many common and unusual diseases.

Chlorella helps to strengthen xue (blood), chi (vitality, energy) and Chen (soul).

This is very important for maintaining a healthy body.

As example, many people can notice increased energy levels, that high blood pressure is normalized and that need for sweetener decreases.

Many vitamin supplements on the market can contain synthetic constituents e.g. as vitamin C in synthetic form, that in most cases, contain artificial ingredients and has no bioenergy (chi, qi) like vitamin in chlorella has.

Other green products like spirulina, wheat grass and barley lacking chlorella's cell wall and CGF (Chlorella Growth Factor) are completely different chlorella and do not, in all, possess the same property as chlorella.

Chlorella can be used as a preventive nutrition, a means for better body balance and stimulus for normalizing the body's functions and constitutes of a healing, revitalizing, rejuvenating and anti-aging food.

SOME GOOD PIECES OF ADVICE!

Do not fry or use heated oil when frying. When roasting, nutritional values are reduced in the food and lecithin is destroyed which is necessary for the fat balance and makes the food more easy to assimilate.

The temperature in food that occurs when cooking and frying in oil changes the nutritional chemistry, which is not reliable. One of the main contributing causes of unhealthy cholesterol formation risking arterial and cardiovascular disease is the use of oils and greases when boiled or overcooked (100 c).

2.

Do not eat until you feel the harmonious balance of mind and body and are free from stress. We do not burn the food well if we are upset or when we are not in good balance.

3.

Do not eat until you feel hungry. Too often, we eat just because it's food time, not because we feel hunger.

4. Eat only as much as you need to eat and avoid becoming over-saturated.

Chew your food thoroughly, which facilitates combustion. **We eat to build health.** You need food that can meet the need for an active life and the following nutritional rules are designed for just this purpose. These are physical laws that can be used. Food should be natural and pure.

Explanation: Food supplement from nature that is 100% organic detects genetics in body and take up the nutrient content more efficiently.

Some foods such as potatoes, root crops and cereals must be prepared.

6. We should daily eat 60 raw foods.

 I suggest raw food (vegetables, fruit) because I think it's more useful for us.
Raw food contributes to more vitamins, minerals, enzymes and fiber because it is "live" food with optimal nutritional value if it is well chosen.
We should eat six vegetables, two fruits, one starch and one protein every day to get the right and balanced nutritional intake.
Vegetables are rich in fiber and minerals. Fruits contain a natural complex of sugar and vitamins. Starch is the energy and protein for cell repair and reconstruction, especially for the brain and nerves. To keep the body in good balance, we need to eat 60-80% alkaline food food and 20-40% acid producing food.

(Dietary fats are actually the preferred fuel of human metabolism, and this can be traced back to our evolutionary roots.
One of the keys to long-term weight management and good health is healthy mitochondrial function and for that you need to get your net carb, protein and fat ratios correct).
Explanation: 80% of the nutrients injected with the blood are alkaline and 20% acid-forming.
 In order to achieve a good blood balance, 6 vegetables and 2 fruits represent the 80% baseline food we need, while 1 protein and 1 starch contribute to the 20% acidic-formation we need. Variation: Varying proteins, starches, vegetables and fruits from meal to meal, and day by day.
Explanation: Every organ in the body needs a chemical element more than others to remain healthy.

The thyroid gland needs iodine, the stomach needs sodium, the blood needs iron and so on. We also need vitamin variation.

The best way to accomplish the latter is to vary the diet. Eat moderately. Avoid eating food after a certain pattern involving only a few nutrients.

Explanation: The larger the waist dimensions, the shorter the lifespan.

Abundance of a diet consisting of only a few foods prevents us from receiving a varied vitamin supplement that is necessary to meet the nutritional requirements of the body.

Combination: Separate starch and protein.

Explanation: Use protein and starches at separate meals, not because they can't be melted well together, but to allow more fruits and vegetables to be consumed at each meal. People generally seem to fill up the meal with protein and starch and avoid vegetables. Be careful of drinking tap water.

Explanation: Most water systems are treated with chemicals because the groundwater is exposed more and more to pollution. Please use an suitable filter.

Reduce the intake of carbohydrates such as sweets, pasta, potatoes, rice, crackers, cookies, sugar and bread.

Think of the body's insulin and glucose balance. Exercise more, preferably every day at least an hour and above all outdoors.

Please feel free to walk with acceleration and learn to breathe correctly.

In stressful work, you should give yourself 5 minutes of relaxation every hour with the help of meditation and muscle relaxation.
Try to think positively about your everyday life and your environment and turn negative thoughts into positive thoughts.

Sleep is necessary and it is important to get a deep sleep (grade 4) Remember to try to go to bed before 22.00 hour.
The beneficial bacteria found in fermented foods have been shown particularly effective for suppressing colon cancer, but may also inhibit cancers of the breast, liver, small intestine and other organs.

Your immune system is the first line of defense; a weakened immune system is what allows diseases such as cancer. Reducing inflammation is a foundational aspect of cancer prevention.

Drink at least two litters of water every day. Water should be consumed in small portions during the day. Avoid drinking water after 18.00 hour.

Since today's food does not contain enough nutrition, one needs to eat a dietary supplement that is complete, well balanced and preferably in 100% organic natural form without additives of binders or synthetic substances.
The body recognizes the nutrient and absorbs it more effectively than than when taking synthetic drugs. Chlorella pyrenoidosa is a good and fully nutritious food as example.

Try to keep a more basic environment in your body. Avoid eating foods that acidify the body too much. It is important with the acid/base balance.
If possible, avoid antibiotics and other drugs. Only in cases of absolute emergency and after medical advice, medicines should be used.

Use a natural probiotics that assist your own good bacteria and strengthens them in the fight against foreign bacteria and heavy metals. Chlorella is an effective probiotics.
Make sure your stomach works with good bowel movements daily and at least once a day. Express your feelings because repressed feelings are as stressful to the body as other types of trauma and poisoning processes.

Encourage the body to fight the free radicals by eating nutritious foods with protective antioxidants.
Today, supplements are needed because nutrition in our daily foods does not contain enough antioxidants.
Carotene (vitamin A), vitamin C, vitamin E, selenium, chromium, zinc, folic acid and vitamin B12 are powerful antioxidants.
There has recently been said that antioxidants do not protect us against colon cancer and other cancerous diseases. It is also said that too much antioxidants can instead constitute a risk of cancer. I'm sure there are synthetically produced antioxidants that are meant and not those found in vegetables and fruits and in 100% organic, non-man-made plants.

The only thing that can protect us from different forms of cancer is a human-adapted lifestyle that allows the body to maintain a good balance of function.

To achieve this, it is important to eat properly and otherwise take care of the body in a sensible way which means, among other things, trying to maintain a strong immune system.

Part of the holistic self-treatment of the body may advantageously consist supplements of vitamins, minerals, fatty acids, proteins, enzymes and other important nutrients in a completely 100% natural form as in Chlorella pyrenoidosa.

Because the body is a self-healing organism, it needs daily " proper fuel ".

References

Nakano, S; Takekoshi, H; Nakano, M (2007). "Chlorella (Chlorella pyrenoidosa) supplementation decreases dioxin and increases immunoglobulin a concentrations in breast milk. Journal of Medicinal Food. **10** (1): 134–42. doi: 10.1089/jmf.2006.023. PMID 17472477.
•

Bovee, H H; Pilgrim, A J; Sun, L S; Schubert, J E; Eng, T L; Benishek, B J. "Large Algal Systems" (PDF). Contrails. Illinois Institute of Technology. p. 12.
• Merchant, R. E.; Andre, C. A. (2001). "A review orecent clinical trials of the nutritional supplement Chlorella pyrenoidosa in the treatment of fibromyalgia, hypertension, and ulcerative colitis". Alternative therapies in health and medicine.
• **7** (3): 79–91. PMID 11347287.

*Boraas, M. E. 1983. Predator induced evolution in chemostat culture. EOS. Transaction of the American Geophysical Union. 64:1102.

• Watanabe F, et al Characterization of a vitamin B12 compound in the edible purple laver, Porphyra yezoensis . Biosci Biotechnol Biochem. (2000)

• Takenaka S, et al Feeding dried purple laver (nori) to vitamin B12-deficient rats significantly improves vitamin B12 status . Br J Nutr. (2001)

• Miyamoto E, et al Characterization of a vitamin B12 compound from unicellular coccolithophorid alga (Pleurochrysis carterae) . J Agric Food Chem. (2001)

• Rauma AL, et al Vitamin B-12 status of long-term adherents of a strict uncooked vegan diet ("living food diet") is compromised . J Nutr. (1995)

• Wawrik B, Harriman BH Rapid, colorimetric quantification of lipid from algal cultures . J Microbiol Methods. Biodiesel from microalgae.

• Park JY1, et al Changes in fatty acid composition of Chlorella vulgaris by hypochlorous acid. Bioresour Technol. (2014)

• Mišurcová L1, et al Amino acid composition of algal products and its contribution to RDI . Food Chem. (2014)

• Kittaka-Katsura H, et al Purification and characterization of a corrinoid compound from Chlorella tablets as an algal health food . J Agric Food Chem. (2002)

• Watanabe F, et al Characterization and bioavailability of vitamin B12-compounds from edible algae . J Nutr Sci Vitaminol (Tokyo). (2002)

• Uchikawa T, et al Chlorella suppresses methylmercury transfer to the fetus in pregnant mice . J Toxicol Sci. (2011)

• Tamaki H, et al Inhibitory effects of herbal extracts on breast cancer resistance protein (BCRP) and structure-inhibitory potency relationship of isoflavonoids . Drug Metab Pharmacokinet. (2010)

• Rai UN1, et al Chromate tolerance and accumulation in Chlorella vulgaris L.: role of antioxidant enzymes and biochemical changes in detoxification of metals . Bioresour Technol. (2013)

• Algal Biomass: An Economical Method for Removal of Chromium from Tannery Effluent

• Jiang Y1, et al Effects of arsenate (AS5+) on growth and production of glutathione (GSH) and phytochelatins (PCS) in Chlorella vulgaris . Int J Phytoremediation. (2011)

- Karadjova IB1, Slaveykova VI, Tsalev DL The biouptake and toxicity of arsenic species on the green microalga Chlorella salina in seawater . Aquat Toxicol. (2008)
- Wu Y1, Wang WX Accumulation, subcellular distribution and toxicity of inorganic mercury and methylmercury in marine phytoplankton . Environ Pollut. (2011)

- Uchikawa T, et al Enhanced elimination of tissue methylmercury in Parachlorella beijerinckii-fed mice . J Toxicol Sci. (2011)
- Uchikawa T, et al The influence of Parachlorella beyerinckii CK-5 on the absorption and excretion of methylmercury (MeHg) in mice . J Toxicol Sci. (2010)
- The Prevalence of Anemia in Women

- Kusumi E, et al Prevalence of anemia among healthy women in 2 metropolitan areas of Japan . Int J Hematol. (2006)
- Matsuura E, et al Effect of chlorella on rats with iron deficient anemia . Kitasato Arch Exp Med. (1991)

- Nakano S, Takekoshi H, Nakano M Chlorella pyrenoidosa supplementation reduces the risk of anemia, proteinuria and edema in pregnant women . Plant Foods Hum Nutr. (2010)

- Shimada M, et al Anti-hypertensive effect of gamma-aminobutyric acid (GABA)-rich Chlorella on high-normal blood pressure and borderline hypertension in placebo-controlled double blind study . Clin Exp Hypertens. (2009)

- Lee SH, et al Six-week supplementation with Chlorella has favorable impact on antioxidant status in Korean male smokers . Nutrition. (2010)

- Nakashima Y, et al Preventive effects of Chlorella on cognitive decline in age-dependent dementia model mice . Neurosci Lett. (2009)

• Mizoguchi T, et al Nutrigenomic studies of effects of Chlorella on subjects with high-risk factors for lifestyle-related disease . J Med Food. (2008)

• Merchant RE, Carmack CA, Wise CM Nutritional supplementation with Chlorella pyrenoidosa for patients with fibromyalgia syndrome: a pilot study. Phytother Res. (2000)
• Merchant RE, Andre CA A review of recent clinical trials of the nutritional supplement Chlorella pyrenoidosa in the treatment of fibromyalgia, hypertension, and ulcerative colitis . Altern Ther Health Med. (2001)

• Otsuki T, et al Salivary secretory immunoglobulin A secretion increases after 4-weeks ingestion of chlorella-derived multicomponent supplement in humans: a randomized cross over study . Nutr J. (2011)

• Lamm ME, et al IgA and mucosal defense . APMIS. (1995)

   • Klentrou P, et al Effect of moderate exercise on salivary immunoglobulin A and infection risk in humans . Eur J Appl Physiol. (2002)

• Gleeson M, et al Salivary IgA levels and infection risk in elite swimmers . Med Sci Sports Exerc. (1999)

• Nakano S, Takekoshi H, Nakano M Chlorella (Chlorella pyrenoidosa) supplementation decreases dioxin and increases immunoglobulin a concentrations in breast milk . J Med Food. (2007)

• Halperin SA, et al Safety and immunoenhancing effect of a Chlorella-derived dietary supplement in healthy adults undergoing influenza vaccination: randomized, double-blind, placebo-controlled trial . CMAJ. (2003)

• Lai KM, Scrimshaw MD, Lester JN Biotransformation and bioconcentration of steroid estrogens by Chlorella vulgaris . Appl Environ Microbiol. (2002)

- Ge L, et al Photodegradation of 17beta-estradiol induced by Chlorella vulgaris . Ying Yong Sheng Tai Xue Bao. (2004)

- Hirooka T, et al Biodegradation of bisphenol A and disappearance of its estrogenic activity by the green alga Chlorella fusca var. vacuolata. Environ Toxicol Chem. (2005)

- Nakano S, Takekoshi H, Nakano M Chlorella pyrenoidosa supplementation reduces the risk of anemia, proteinuria and edema in pregnant women
- Plant Foods Hum Nutr. (2010)

- Lee SH, et al Six-week supplementation with Chlorella has favorable impact on antioxidant status in Korean male smokers . Nutrition. (2010)

- Otsuki T, et al Salivary secretory immunoglobulin A secretion increases after 4-weeks ingestion of chlorella-derived multicomponent supplement in humans: a randomized cross over study. Nutr J. (2011)

- Shimada M, et al Anti-hypertensive effect of gamma-aminobutyric acid (GABA)-rich Chlorella on high-normal blood pressure and borderline hypertension in placebo-controlled double blind study. Clin Exp Hypertens. (2009)

- Halperin SA, et al Safety and immunoenhancing effect of a Chlorella-derived dietary supplement in healthy adults undergoing influenza vaccination: randomized, double-blind, placebo-controlled trial. CMAJ. (2003)

- Merchant RE, Carmack CA, Wise CM Nutritional supplementation with Chlorella pyrenoidosa for patients with fibromyalgia syndrome: a pilot study. Phytother Res. (2000) American Institute of Chemical Engineers Biotechnol. Prog., 2013.

Chlorella pyrenoidosa is a unicellular green algae and has been a popular foodstuff worldwide. However, no reports on the anti tumor peptides from such a micro algae are available in the literature.

• Halperin SA, et al Safety and immunoenhancing effect of a Chlorella-derived dietary supplement in healthy adults undergoing influenza vaccination: randomized, double-blind, placebo-controlled trial. CMAJ. (200

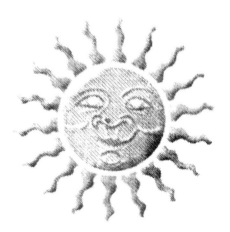

Stig Arne Levin

CHLORELLA
-FUNCTIONAL FOOD-

Copyright: Stig A. Levin © 2018
ISBN 978-0-244-38980-2

Cover design: Caussimon Pascal, France

Made in the USA
Monee, IL
29 June 2022